P9-APR-396

Praise for
Nick Littlehales and *Sleep*

"Nick Littlehales wants to redefine the very meaning of the word 'sleep.'"

—*Daily Telegraph*

"Nick Littlehales has reconfigured the bedrooms of a legion of international sporting stars. . . . He has a unique and encyclopedic knowledge."

—*Guardian*

"Sleep guru Nick Littlehales trains elite athletes to get the best possible rest."

—*Daily Mail*

"This is a tremendously exciting development and one I wholeheartedly support. Nick Littlehales provides leading professionals in the world of sport, including Manchester United, with a better understanding of this natural physical and mental process—he enables players to maximize the quality and consistency of their sleep and in turn their overall performance."

—Alex Ferguson, former manager, Manchester United Football Club

"Nick has revolutionized my recovery process through practical, tailored professional advice."

—Helen Wyman, European Cyclocross champion

"Nick Littlehales is an innovative, world-class thinker. He designed the sleep solution for Team Sky's riders—who have now won the Tour de France four times—and British Cycling, who have used his principles of sleep optimization at the last two Olympics to great effect."

—Philip Burt, lead physical therapist, British Cycling

SLEEP

SLEEP

The Myth of 8 Hours, the Power of Naps . . .
and the New Plan to Recharge Your Body and Mind

NICK LITTLEHALES

Da Capo

LIFE
LONG

Note: The information in this book is true and complete to the best of our knowledge. This book is intended only as an informative guide for those wishing to know more about health issues. In no way is this book intended to replace, countermand, or conflict with the advice given to you by your own physician. The ultimate decision concerning care should be made between you and your doctor. We strongly recommend you follow his or her advice. Information in this book is general and is offered with no guarantees on the part of the authors or Da Capo Press. The authors and publisher disclaim all liability in connection with the use of this book. The names and identifying details of certain people associated with events described in this book have been changed. Any similarity to actual persons is coincidental.

Copyright © 2017 by Nick Littlehales

Hachette Book Group supports the right to free expression and the value of copyright. The purpose of copyright is to encourage writers and artists to produce the creative works that enrich our culture.

The scanning, uploading, and distribution of this book without permission is a theft of the author's intellectual property. If you would like permission to use material from the book (other than for review purposes), please contact permissions@hbgusa.com. Thank you for your support of the author's rights.

Da Capo Lifelong Books
Hachette Book Group
1290 Avenue of the Americas
New York, NY 10104
www.dacapopress.com
@dacapopress

Printed in the United States of America

Originally published in 2016 by Penguin Life in the United Kingdom

First US edition: March 2018

Published by Da Capo Press, an imprint of Perseus Books, LLC, a subsidiary of Hachette Book Group, Inc. The Da Capo Lifelong name and logo is a trademark of the Hachette Book Group.

The publisher is not responsible for websites (or their content) that are not owned by the publisher.

ISBNs: 978-0-7382-3462-5 (paperback); 978-0-7382-3463-2 (ebook)

LSC-C

10 9 8 7 6 5 4 3 2 1

For my father, Herbert James Littlehales

Contents

Introduction

Don't Waste Your Valuable Time Sleeping

When I asked the person behind the counter of my local bookstore where the sleep section was, she gave me a quizzical look, turned to her computer, and, after some searching, pointed me in what she hoped was the right direction. Up four flights of stairs, in a dark and dusty corner, I finally found it: a small collection of academic tomes on the science of sleep, plus a handful of volumes on dreams and what they mean—New Age takes on an age-old process.

My hope is that this is not where you found this book.

There is a revolution going on in sleep. For too long it has been an aspect of our lives that we take for granted, and historical patterns suggest we've placed less and less importance on sleep itself (certainly by leaving fewer hours for it). But a burgeoning body of scientific research is drawing links between our poor sleeping habits and an array of health and psychological issues, from type 2 diabetes, heart disease, and obesity to anxiety and burnout. It's time for sleep to take its place in the spotlight. It's time to look at this essential process of mental and physical recovery and see how we can do it better, so that we can get the most out of our waking day and be more effective at work, give our best to our relationships with family and friends, and feel great.

Until the mid-1990s we were getting away with it. Most of us took for granted that we'd get two consecutive days off (otherwise known as the weekend). Our work finished when we left the office—or wherever it was we did our jobs—and many stores were closed on Sundays. Then came a seismic change in our lifestyle. The Internet and email altered forever the way we communicate, consume, and work, and mobile phones, initially just devices for phone calls and texting, soon morphed into the little pools of blue light at which we now spend so much of our time gazing. The idea of being constantly connected became a reality, the 24/7 working mentality was born, and we had to make adjustments to keep up. Overstimulating on caffeine, popping sleeping pills to come down and switch off, burning the candle at both ends—the traditional idea of a good eight hours' sleep at night became the stuff of legend.

The result has been extra stresses and strains on relationships and family life. Not only that, some scientists and researchers connect our lack of physical and mental recovery time with a tangible increase in many diseases and disorders. Something has to give.

I am a sports sleep coach. It's a job that is unlikely to come up at your local career center, and that's largely because it's a role I've managed to create for myself.

This journey began when I was the international sales and marketing director of Slumberland, the largest sleeping comfort group in Europe, in the late 1990s. I became intrigued by what the top soccer team in the country did about sleep and recovery. *They must have a sophisticated approach to it all*, I thought, so I wrote to Manchester United, a club now owned by the Glazer family (who also own the Tampa Bay Buccaneers NFL franchise), to find out. It turned out that they did nothing. The reply from Manchester United manager Alex Ferguson—who would soon make history by leading the club to unprecedented levels of success—asked if I'd be interested in coming in and taking a look.

Sleep wasn't considered a performance factor back then, but I was fortunate that sports science was becoming a bigger part of the game and that the curiosity of one of the greatest managers of all time had been piqued. I was equally fortunate that I was able to work with a player who had a back problem, and we made some adjustments to his routine and products. You can't cure a back injury with a mattress, of course, no matter what some manufacturers might claim, but I was able to have a positive impact on the player's management of his condition.

I became more heavily involved with the club, even providing Ferguson with some products and advice, as well as some of the most famous players, including David Beckham and Ryan Giggs. This top-down approach, where everyone from the manager and coaching staff to the players uses the methods and products I've recommended, is one I implement to this day.

By this time I was in the process of leaving my role at Slumberland. The world of sleep had begun to engage me beyond simply selling products. I had been chairman of the UK Sleep Council, a consumer education organization set up to advise on and promote better sleep quality, which helped further my knowledge, and it was there that I got to know Chris Idzikowski, a leading expert in the field, who would grow to be a valued friend and colleague. Meanwhile, the press had coined my job title, branding me Manchester United's "sleep coach." "What's he doing," they asked, "tucking the players in at night?" In fact, I was doing things like introducing probably the first training-facility sleep recovery room on the planet. Lots of top teams have them now, of course, but that was the first.

Word spread. The Manchester United players on England's national team competing in the World Cup and European Championship soon had English Football Association executives and physical therapists coming my way. I worked with the organization, having new sleeping products shipped in and advising players on improving their habits. And I began working with several other teams, who were responding to new sports science and changing their approach to the game. Later, I would work with British Cycling and Team Sky, including their successful Tour de France campaigns. I designed portable sleep kits for the riders to sleep on instead of the beds in their hotel rooms. I would be brought in by British Olympians and Paralympians and by athletes in sports such as rowing, sailing, bobsled, BMX, and cyclocross, as well as by rugby and cricket teams and many more soccer clubs.

This revolution in the sporting world wasn't confined to Britain; sleep is universal, after all. I was invited to join up with leading European soccer clubs such as Real Madrid, where I advised on adapting their luxury training-facility player apartments into the ideal recovery rooms for some of the world's best players. I worked with the Dutch women's bobsled team before the Winter Olympics in 2014, and I coach cyclists from places as far away as Malaysia.

I have brought my methods to the United States too, teaming up with SHIFT Performance to work with teams like the NFL's Miami Dolphins and some of the leading colleges around the country, and I've had conversations with people like Tim DiFrancesco, the former LA Lakers basketball strength and conditioning coach, about giving the leading athletes in the sport the best chance of recovery. The amount of travel involved in many sports thanks to the size of the United States and the stresses that games like football put on the bodies of the players present new and unique challenges to their ability to recover properly.

All of this came about because I was the first to ask the professional sporting world about sleep, and because Alex Ferguson, whose willingness to embrace new ideas never dimmed during his decades at the top of his sport, was sufficiently open-minded to help me explore the subject. As he said at the time, "This is a tremendously exciting development in the world of sport, and one I wholeheartedly support."

The reaction of many people when they hear what I do is to conjure up images of sleek sleep pods and high-tech science-fiction-style white labs with slumbering subjects wired up to supercomputers, but nothing could be further from the truth. Yes, I use all sorts of technology when necessary, and yes, I've worked closely with leading academics in the field of sleep such as Idzikowski, but my day-to-day work isn't in a laboratory or a clinic—I'm not a doctor or a scientist.

In recent years, the importance of sleep for our health has been proven with clinical evidence. Revered institutions around the world—Harvard, Stanford, Oxford, and the University of Munich, among many others—produce pioneering research in the field. This research has demonstrated everything from the links between sleep and obesity and diabetes[1] to showing that our brains effectively wash away their waste toxins during sleep, potentially illuminating one of the key reasons we sleep.[2] Failure to get enough sleep and clear out these toxins is linked to a host of neurological disorders, including Alzheimer's.

The health factor is a big reason why governments and businesses are starting to prick up their ears and listen when it comes to sleep, and why more attention is being given to re-search and funding. Stress and burnout are bad for business.

But as mind-bendingly smart as the people researching sleep are, there's so much about sleep that we just haven't yet figured out. As Philippe Mourrain, associate professor at the Stanford Center for Sleep Sciences and Medicine, writes, "We don't really know what sleep is. This may come as a shock to the uninitiated."

What we *do* know—and even the scientists can all agree on this—is that sleep is vital to our well-being. Quite simply, we're not getting enough of it. It is estimated that, on average, we're getting between one and two hours *less* sleep than we were in the 1950s.[3] So, is the answer that we should simply get more of it?

What about a single parent who is up at the crack of dawn to get the kids off to school, works all day, and then comes home at night to make dinner, put the children to bed, and then get the housework done before collapsing into bed? How is that person supposed to fit more sleep in? Or a medical resident working all the hours that the job entails, as well as trying to maintain some faint sliver of a personal life—how is it possible for them to get more sleep? There are only so many hours in the day. How does sleep research directly benefit their lives? What can everyday people take from it beyond an interesting nugget of information they might read in the news on the train to work and forget about by the time they sit down at their desks?

Athletes, whose activities during most of their waking hours are already subject to intensive scrutiny from college and professional coaches who want them to perform at their absolute best when they're on the field, don't want too much of a clinical approach to their sleep. After all, sleep is one of the few remaining privacies we have, away from the glare of our employers, who have managed to enter our personal lives through our phones. People generally don't want to be wired up and monitored while they sleep, with the truth about what they're up to at night being shared with their supervisors at work. It's too intrusive.

My approach is different. Science and research inform what I do, of course, but I'm hands-on, working directly with people to give them the maximum advantages in recovery so that they can perform at their best when it matters. What I see, and the people who apply my methods to their lives see, is a vast improvement in the way they feel, in the way they recover, and, most important, in their level of performance. This is the benchmark clinical test for any professional athlete, and there's no arguing with the empirical results that competitive sports provide.

I talk to these performers about their habits, give them practical advice, and arm them with the skills to plan and manage their rest in clinically accepted cycles of sleep. I design and source their sleeping products, help them with everything from coping with a newborn in the family to getting them off sleeping pills; ensure hotel rooms are producing a conducive environment for recovery for cyclists on the tour and soccer players at international tournaments; and, when needed, go into their homes and address their sleeping setups there.

However, for those of you hoping for a sleep-and-tell exposé on the contents of David Beckham's bedside table, you're in for a disappointment. These performers and sporting institutions trust me implicitly. They're letting me into a very personal and private sanctuary, and I've had to earn that right. After all, would you let someone you didn't trust into your bedroom? But what I *can* tell you all about is the methods and techniques I bring into these sanctuaries, and I can show you how to set up yours just like an elite athlete.

Fine, you might be thinking, *but what do the sleep habits of top athletes have to do with me?* The simple answer is absolutely everything. All of the advice and techniques outlined in this book are as relevant to you or me as they are to the players. Indeed, I work with many people outside of sports, from corporate clients to anyone looking to improve their sleep regimen at home. The only difference between top athletes and the rest of us in this regard is quite simple: *commitment.* If I tell an Olympic athlete what to do to improve their recovery, they do it. Sports people are like that. If they can see a gain to be made, no matter how marginal, they'll go for it, because it all adds up and they're in the business of performing better than their opponents. For the rest of us, it's all too easy to adhere to a method for a few days before real life starts intervening, and next thing we know we're working well into the night or passing out on the sofa after a few too many glasses of wine.

But this book isn't a fad "sleep diet." I'm not going to give you a rigid scheme to stick to that you'll abandon after a week. I don't want to make your life more difficult. I am going to show you my R90 Sleep Recovery Program, the very method I use with elite athletes. I have developed this program over nearly two decades as a professional sleep coach, acquiring knowledge from doctors, academics, sports scientists, physiotherapists, mattress and bedding manufacturers, and even my children, through the experience of being a parent. I've tested my methods at the forefront of professional sports, where sleep simply must be effective. These athletes operate at the margins of what is possible for human beings to achieve, and I can show you how you can work at the margins of what is possible for you too.

Through integrating this approach into your own life, you will be able to reap the benefits of the extra mental and physical energy you will feel. You will learn to look at sleeping in a polyphasic way. I will help you choose the best sleeping position (and there is only one that I recommend). You will no longer think about how many hours a night you're sleeping; rather, you'll think in terms of how many *cycles per week* you're fitting in. This will help you learn to accept and relax about the odd bad night's sleep—we all have them, and we all get up in the morning and carry on.

It will inform your decisions about things in your day-to-day life that you might never have thought about before: which desk to sit at in an office, choosing a side of the bed in a hotel with a partner, or whether the bedroom in the house you're considering buying is fit for the purpose (and if it's not, that should be a deal-breaker). I will set out the seven Key Sleep Recovery Indicators, which are the building blocks of the R90 program. Within each of these I will give you seven steps to improve your sleep. Even adopting just one of them could go a long way toward improving your life. And if you adopt one per week, you can completely revolutionize your sleep in just seven weeks.

Your lifestyle won't have to suffer. You can still have that inviting-looking coffee you crave. You don't have to say no to another glass of wine when you're enjoying a fine summer night with friends. And if you're sitting down to dinner in a restaurant after nine o'clock and wondering if it's too late to be eating, don't worry. Life's too short to miss out on good times and great experiences. I want to give you the confidence to make these decisions and have the flexibility not to worry about getting to bed "on time" or stress about "sleeping well." Through adopting the measures mapped out in this book, you can learn to improve the *quality* of your rest and recovery, rather than spend time agonizing over the quantity.

This book will explain what we can learn from our Paleolithic ancestors to better regulate our sleep—think a Paleo *sleep* diet—while also managing modern-day challenges like smart-phones, laptops, jet lag, and working late. Technology is a won-derful thing, and I certainly won't be advocating discarding it just to get a good night's sleep—all of our devices are here to stay, and this is only the beginning of it—but with just a little more awareness on our part, they don't have to be detrimental to our well-being.

We'll see how your love life can dramatically improve with just a little bedroom know-how, why we should all hail the power of the afternoon nap—and how you can nap with your eyes wide open in a room full of people. I'm going to show you that, in all likelihood, the mattress you're sleeping on is the wrong one, even—or maybe especially—if it's a $2,000 "ortho-pedic" slab you've just remortgaged your house for. The good news is that I can show you how it doesn't have to cost an arm and a leg to remedy it. I will give you a foolproof method for picking the right surface to sleep on that will mean you'll never again have to endure another salesperson trying to sell you a multi-thousand-coil mattress with racing stripes and a price tag to match.

The R90 Sleep Recovery Program shares some of the spirit of Team Sky performance director Dave Brailsford's "aggregation of marginal gains" approach. With the cycling team, recruit-ing my expertise in sleep was just one of many ways in which Brailsford sought to make a tiny improvement (another was teaching the riders the best way to wash their hands in order to avoid catching a virus), so that when they were all added up it would produce a significant increase in performance.

With the R90 approach, we look at everything we do from waking until closing our eyes at night as having an effect on our sleep. As we funnel our attention down toward going to bed, we can aggregate our own marginal gains by implementing the advice set out in the Key Sleep Recovery Indicators.

You might not see results overnight—even after a partic-ularly good night's sleep. But give it time. It usually takes pro-fessional athletes years to reach the top of their sport. You'll see results in your sleep much quicker than that with the R90 program. It's not uncommon for me to receive a call from someone a few months after we've worked together and hear them say, "You changed my life."

You can change yours too. Let's start using the time you spend asleep wisely. Like the athletes I work with, you should be getting the absolute maximum of physical and mental recovery out of it. You might learn that you actually need *less* sleep. You will certainly feel an improvement in your mood and capabilities at work and at home, and you'll also become more aware of when it's time to pull back a little, to take a break and switch off for a few minutes. "Oh, but I don't have time for that," you're saying. Think again. There is a host of little tricks and techniques to find time for breaks, enabling you to get more done in less time.

If you want a book about how to get your pajamas on and have a cozy time in bed with your cocoa, then you've come to the wrong place, though I can certainly point you in the direction of a dusty corner. I am, however, going to show you how to sleep smarter, to use sleep as a natural mental and physical performance enhancer. It's time to stop wasting time on sleeping without benefit.

PART ONE

The Key Sleep Recovery Indicators

ONE

The Clock Is Ticking

Circadian Rhythms

You wake up to the alarm on your phone and reach over to turn it off. While you're there, you check the notifications beamed in overnight from your news, sports, and entertainment feeds, your social media apps, emails and texts from work and friends. Your mouth is dry, your head is already spinning with what's to come this morning, the curtains are leaking light, and the standby light on the TV at the foot of the bed is staring unblinkingly at you, reminding you how you finished the night before.

Welcome to your day. Did you sleep well? Do you know *how* to sleep well?

The average person in the United States gets a little over six and a half hours of sleep a night. Furthermore, over a quarter of the population gets by on only six hours a night, and 14 percent get five hours or less.[1] It's a similar story around the world, with over a third of the population of Britain reporting less than six hours of sleep on workdays, and Japan not far behind. The statistics show that in these countries, as well as the likes of

Canada and Germany, most people "catch up" on their sleep on the weekend.[2] Their work lives are limiting their sleep. Almost half of Americans are being kept awake by stress or worry, and when you take a look at the schedules of many people, it's not difficult to see why.[3]

An NBA athlete might compete in a game on the West Coast one day and then be back across the country the next day to hear me talk to the team about sleep. He's probably wondering when he's supposed to get any, as he's about to spend the next few months on the road, playing in games all over the United States. You can do it for a while, of course, with the right approach. Round-the-world solo sailors can get by sleeping for thirty minutes every twelve hours while they're at sea for three months; we're remarkably adaptable creatures with incredible reserves of stamina. But do it for too long, and sooner or later something has to give. Sports associations are starting to bring me in to educate players and help them manage their schedules, because they're seeing a rise in the number of players coming to them with depression, relationship problems, and burnout.

It's not just in sports, of course. These patterns are replicated all over society. All of us face difficulties fitting in the demands of our work and personal lives. Knowing what I know now, I can say that I stayed in a job for five years too long. I was working long hours, with an abundance of day-to-day stress and plenty of travel, which meant a lot of time away from home. But they were business-class trips along with plenty of fine dining, gin and tonics, and coffee to keep me going, so at the time I thought I could handle it. The truth is that it took a very heavy toll on my family life.

How much was I sleeping then? How much are players on the US national soccer team getting? What about that teenager sitting up playing computer games deep into the night? How much are you sleeping? Does it actually matter?

The amount isn't the important thing at this stage. What is important is a natural process that has been with us since humankind began, a process that many of the aspects of modern life are taking us away from. Artificial light, technology, shift work, sleeping pills, travel, checking our phones when we wake, working late, even running out of the house and skipping breakfast to race to our jobs on time—all these things are taking us away from this natural process. And that's where our problems with rest and recovery begin.

Off the Grid

Let's start by going off the grid for a while. Let's get back to nature for real. You and I will leave all our possessions behind—our watches, computers, phones—and head out to an uninhabited island, where we'll live off the land, just as our ancestors once did. We'll hunt and fish and sleep under the stars. Eat your heart out, Bear Grylls.

So out there on this island we make camp in a large rolling field. When the sun eventually goes down, and the temperature drops with it, we build a fire. We're going to spend quite a lot of time now without daylight, so we want to eat. We cook and devour our spoils for the day, and then sit back sated, chatting softly, absorbing the amber light of the fire as we look into it. Eventually the talk subsides, and we gaze up at the stars for a while before, one by one, we turn over, curl up under our blankets, and drift off into sleep.

At some point in the morning, the sun is going to start approaching the horizon. The birds will start singing even before it gets there, and when it does, the temperature will start to rise. Even if it's really cold, it will still rise by a degree or two, and everything will get lighter. Whether or not we've got our heads under the blankets, the light gets in and we wake up. The first thing we're likely to want to do is empty our bladders, and then we'll start thinking about drinking some water and eating breakfast. Then it'll be time for a bowel movement before we go fishing and hunting and gathering for the day—all of it in daylight. Nothing hurried, all in its natural time.

Later in the day, when the sun starts going down again, we'll sit back down in the field. The temperature will drop and it will get dark again, so we'll have to light the fire—we'll do it all again. This is really getting back to what we do naturally, working in harmony with our circadian rhythms.

Got Rhythm?

One of the first things I ask anyone I work with, whether it's a top athlete or a corporate executive struggling to sleep, is, "Are you aware of circadian rhythms?"

A circadian rhythm is a twenty-four-hour internal cycle managed by our body clock. This clock of ours, deep within the brain, regulates our internal systems such as sleeping and eating patterns, hormone production, temperature, alertness, mood, and digestion, in a twenty-four-hour process that evolved to work in harmony with the Earth's rotation. Our body clocks are set by external cues, chief among them being daylight, as well as things like temperature and eating times.

It is vital to understand that these rhythms are ingrained within us; they are part of the fabric of each and every one of us. They are the product of millions of years of evolution. We could no more unlearn these rhythms than we could teach dogs to stop barking or ask a lion if it wouldn't mind giving vegetarianism a try. Each of these animals, of course, has its own body clock and its own circadian rhythms, just as every other animal and plant does. These rhythms function even without external stimuli. If international events conspired to rain a nuclear apocalypse down on us all and we had to move underground and live in caves without daylight, the rhythms would persist within us.

A typical circadian rhythm, which describes what our body *wants* to do naturally at various points throughout the day, looks like this:

So, on our island, once the sun's gone down and we're sitting around the fire, we can see that melatonin secretion starts.

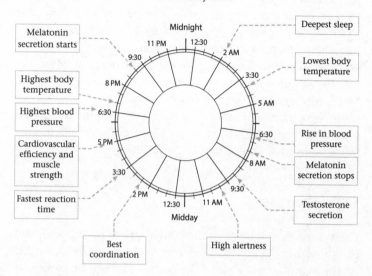

Circadian Rhythms

Melatonin, a hormone that regulates our sleep, is produced in the pineal gland, which responds to light. Once it's been dark for long enough, we produce melatonin to ready ourselves for sleep.

Our body clock isn't the only regulator of our sleep. If we think of circadian rhythms as being our *urge* to sleep, then our homeostatic sleep pressure is our *need* to sleep. This intuitive need builds from the moment we wake up, and the longer we are awake, the greater it becomes. However, our circadian rhythms are able to override this at times, which is why we can experience a "second wind" when we're slumping and why, as many night-shift workers and nightlife lovers will be able to testify, we can have trouble getting to sleep at certain points of the day even if we've been up all night. We're fighting against our body's circadian urge to be up with the sun.

If we keep regular hours and get up in the morning, our need to sleep peaks at night, which coincides with our circadian urge, producing the ideal sleep window. During the night we tend to reach our most effective sleeping period around 2–3 a.m. (which is mirrored by another period of sleepiness twelve hours later, in the form of the midafternoon slump), and our body temperature dips to its lowest point not long after, before the sun comes up and everything gets started again for us. Melatonin secretion stops, just like a switch being flicked, because we're moving from dark to light. Daylight gets our bodies started on producing serotonin, the mood-boosting neurotransmitter from which melatonin is derived.

Light the Way

Light is the most important time setter for our body clocks, and there's nothing better than daylight in the morning for it. Out on the island, sleeping under the sky, we'd get our fix as soon as we woke. But too many of us in the real world spend our time indoors—at home, on the train, in our places of work—and even an overcast day dwarfs any artificial light in terms of brightness. Open the curtains when you wake, eat breakfast and get ready in daylight, and then go outside.

We are particularly sensitive to a wavelength known as blue light. Because of its prevalence in the light given off by electronic devices such as computers and smartphones, blue light gets bad press. But in this case it's not so much that it's bad light—only badly timed light. Daylight is full of blue light, and during the day blue light is *good*. It sets the body clock, suppresses melatonin production, and improves alertness and performance.[4]

Once it's dark, however, these are all undesirable qualities. If you're using devices or have the lights blazing late into the night, then it's going to cause problems. It's going to lead to what Chris Idzikowski calls "junk sleep"—disrupted and diminished sleep as our lifestyles and gadgets inhibit the production of melatonin and push our body clocks later.

On the island it was all daylight and darkness. The light from our fire was the only human-created illumination, and the yellows and ambers and reds that fire gives off don't affect melatonin production.

Sitting by the Fire

No matter what we do in our lives, the sun will go down and it will come up again. When we're in harmony with this process, our brain triggers the functions within us to make the events described on the circadian rhythms chart happen. They might not occur at exactly the times on the chart, but your brain and body will want to do them at some time around then.

Many of us only really become conscious of our circadian rhythms if we fly long haul and experience jet lag, which is when our rhythms are out of sync with the local light-dark cycle because we've traveled so fast across time zones. It's a similar story if we work a night shift and our hours are at odds with the light-dark cycle. But being aware of your body clock in your day-to-day life will allow you to begin to understand why you might be feeling lethargic at certain times of the day, and why you might be struggling to fall asleep. And it's not just your sleep that benefits from this knowledge: it's the whole of your waking day.

If you get up and out as quickly as possible in the morning, grabbing snacks and coffee as you jump on the train to work, you're out of step with your rhythms. Back on our island, we weren't in a rush. We'd have breakfast, and, as our bowels are suppressed overnight, we'd go to the toilet—because we don't want to go when we're out finding food for the day.

It's the same on the train. Is it in your interest to need the toilet on a packed commuter train or to suppress the urge unnaturally? It's no coincidence that you will see advertisements for all sorts of digestion-related products—from yogurt drinks to anti-diarrhea medications—on train station platforms. One of the leading brand's tag lines is "Restore your body's natural rhythm." Right message, wrong answer.

If your exercise regimen involves hitting the gym hard in the early evening, be aware of what that means. Your blood pressure is highest at this time, and the kind of sharp increase in blood pressure that intense exercise causes is something you need to know about, especially if you're a bit older. Just ask the BBC's Andrew Marr about that; he blamed his stroke on a high-intensity session on a rowing machine. Get a wearable fitness tracker, take a look, and maybe see if there's a better time to be doing this.

Think about your rhythms when you're using technology. I don't shy away from it (I don't actually live on an island). I use social media as an important part of my business, I have a smartphone, and I'm just as able to be reached anywhere on the phone or by email as the next person. But I do know that if I've been working on my laptop late at night or video-calling a client in a different time zone when it's convenient for them, the artificial light from my computer is going to suppress the natural sleep process. So I won't go to bed right away; I'll put the laptop to one side and stay up for a bit, so that my pineal gland can function efficiently and get on with producing melatonin now that it's dark, just as it wants to.

So much of what we do in our lives today interferes with our circadian rhythms, and there's little to be done about a lot of it. If we have to work shifts or late into the night, then it's often a case of tough luck for us, since we need to get on with it. But if we're aware of our rhythms, we can make sure we're not doing too many things to add to the problem. We don't want to be at war with our own bodies.

As Russell Foster, director of the Sleep and Circadian Neuroscience Institute at the University of Oxford, told the BBC, "We are the supremely arrogant species; we feel we can abandon four billion years of evolution and ignore the fact that we have evolved under a light-dark cycle. What we do as a species, perhaps uniquely, is override the clock. And long-term acting against the clock can lead to serious health problems."

We've had artificial light only since the nineteenth century. Computers and televisions, let alone smartphones and tablets, are mere babies when put against the length of our evolutionary process. We haven't evolved to cope with these things in the way many of us are using them now.

Whatever it is you're doing, I want you to think about the two of us out on our island, in harmony with a biological process as old as mankind. That is our ideal. Every step we make to improve our sleep, no matter how small, needs to be a step toward our sitting by the fire.

CIRCADIAN RHYTHMS:
SEVEN STEPS TO SLEEP SMARTER

1. Get outside! Set your body clock with daylight, not artificial light.

2. Take the time to learn about your rhythms and how they affect you. Engage family and friends too.

3. Know your peaks and troughs. Monitor yourself and compare that to what should be happening naturally—use a wearable fitness tracker to measure.

4. Peak sleeping time is around 2–3 a.m. If you go to bed as the sun comes up, you are fighting against your body clock.

5. Slow down in your mornings. Rushing off from the word go can disrupt your body. Sleep quality is all about what we do from the point of waking.

6. Blue light is badly timed light in the evening—dim it down when you can. Go for red or yellow light, or even candlelight.

7. Picture yourself by the fire on our island. What are you doing right now that is in conflict with this? What are you going to do about it? Plan simple changes to current routines to align yourself better with the circadian rhythms chart.

TWO

Running Fast and Slow

Chronotype

It's late. The lights in the basketball arena bear down on you and the noise from the crowd is deafening as you look over your sweat-soaked yet defiant players. It's game seven of the NBA Finals, and after the coast-to-coast travel with little recovery between some of the closest games in history, it comes down to this: your teams are tied 3–3 in the series, and in the final quarter your team is just two points behind. The opposition almost has the championship in their grasp, but it's not quite over yet. You are the coach—you must make your final roll of the dice.

You have two players of very similar ability sitting on the bench, and you have to choose between them. Player A hasn't been at his best tonight, particularly as the game has gone on, but he's the consummate professional and has certainly put in the effort. This guy would walk through walls for you. Sure, he looks exhausted, but it has been a long night. Player B, however, has done well. He seems sprightly and alert despite the late hour, but something's bugging you about this guy. He's not disciplined. He's regularly late to training in the morning, and when he does get there it's like he sleepwalks through it. Will he crack under the intense pressure of the dying moments of the closest series he's ever played in? Your eyes are telling you he's the right choice, but your head says go with Player A. You go with your head.

In the very last second of the game, Player A receives the ball in a promising position and lines up to take his shot, your team's last chance to tie the score and take the game into over-time. He should make this shot—he's made it in practice a thou-sand times before. As the ball arcs through the air the horn sounds to mark the end of the game. This is it—all or nothing. The ball sails toward the hoop . . .

And hits the rim, bouncing harmlessly away.

Game over.

Owls and Larks

Once upon a time, long before we started to redefine our ap-proach to sleep, we used to talk about there being two kinds of people: owls and larks. Today we ask, "Do you know your chronotype?"

Your chronotype describes your sleeping characteristics—whether you're a morning or evening person. But it doesn't just determine the time you get up and go to bed. It indicates the times that your body wants to perform the functions outlined in the circadian rhythms chart in Chapter 1, which might come as a relief if you looked at that and thought those timings had no bearing on your life. If you're a morning person (an AMer), your body clock is a bit fast, while if you're the evening type (a PMer), your clock's running slow.

Chronotypes are a genetic trait, and I can usually spot them a mile off in people I meet. Do you like staying up and going to bed late? Do you need an alarm to get you up for work in the morning? Are you partial to a nap in the daytime? Do you often skip breakfast? Do you sleep in on your days off? Then it's likely that you're a PMer.

AMers wake naturally, enjoy their breakfast, and love the mornings. They tend not to need an alarm to wake them, they're less likely to feel fatigued during the day, and they go to bed reasonably early.

This variation is usually only at most by a couple of hours either way, not five or six. Very few people have a makeup whereby they naturally want to wake at noon. Even with the curtains drawn and you hiding away in bed, your brain knows that the sun is up. It wants to be up too. Most of us have an idea of our chronotype, but if you're still unsure, the University of Munich Chronotype Questionnaire is a good place to find out.[1]

As children, we tend to exist as AMers, rising early for the day and usually going to bed long before the adults. When we reach adolescence, however, our body clocks switch to run much slower. We have the urge to go to bed later and sleep in longer. Teenagers get bad press, but they're often just doing what their bodies want them to. As we pass the peak of our late-running clocks, at about the age of twenty, our rhythms revert to their genetic type, and they continue to creep earlier as we get older.[2]

The In-Betweeners

There is a third category of chronotype: the in-betweener. Many of us genuinely are in between, but in fact almost all of the population live their lives as in-betweeners, regardless of their real chronotype. With all the entertainment options available— dinner, drinks, a midnight premiere at the movies, streaming a TV show at home ("Just one more episode before bed . . . ")— why should only the PMers get to enjoy staying up late? And a PMer might like sleeping in (indeed, they're genetically predisposed toward it), but they have to be at work at 9 a.m. tomorrow.

So we mask our true chronotypes by using alarm clocks and by overstimulating: being overactive both physically and mentally, and using caffeine and sugar.

Why is it important to know your chronotype? If we were left to our own devices and could get up and go to sleep whenever we wanted, to wake naturally, and to start work at a time of our own choosing, it wouldn't matter very much. But, strangely enough, working cultures have yet to develop with this in mind. Whether you're an AMer or PMer, you still have to get to work at 9 a.m., you still have to be at practice in the morning if you're a basketball player, and in this instance it's the PMers who suffer because they are effectively trying to operate in a time zone that's different from their internal body clock's. "Social jet lag" is an expression that has been coined to describe this.

Because they naturally get up earlier, AMers tend to get tired sooner and go to bed earlier too. This means that, when morning comes around, they will have enjoyed plenty of restorative deep sleep during the peak time of around 2–3 a.m. and they will be in a lighter sleep state as they approach their wake time. They often won't even need the alarm. PMers, on the other hand, will push on later at night, meaning that when morning comes, the alarm often needs to rouse them from an earlier part of sleep (only for the snooze button to be hit repeatedly), and they will spend the rest of the morning playing catch-up. A PMer is likely to lean on caffeine to do this.

Caffeine Highs and Lows

Caffeine is the world's most popular performance-enhancing drug—a neurostimulant with psychoactive properties that fights off fatigue and has proven beneficial effects on alertness, reaction times, concentration, and endurance.[3]

We use caffeine in sports, particularly in cycling, as a legal and safe boost to performance, but we control its use. We give tailor-made doses to athletes at strategic times (for an endurance event, we would give them a dose nearer the start time than for a sprint), and if a rider turns up after having a double espresso with their breakfast, we would take this into account. There is a coffee culture in all levels of cycling, but the professionals are disciplined enough to be familiar with the caffeine content of the brand they're drinking.

Sarah Piampiano, a professional triathlete and Ironman triathlon champion, doesn't even drink caffeine in her everyday life—she only uses it when she competes, in the form of sports gels with a specific amount of caffeine in them, which she takes before and at various stages throughout the race.

I have, however, seen instances of performers in other sports drinking coffee at home, taking caffeine supplements, and even chewing caffeine gum at practice—consuming it in quantities that are going to have a detrimental effect.

High doses of caffeine can cause agitation and anxiety. Having it in your blood can make it more difficult to get to sleep and more difficult to remain asleep. It is a habit-forming drug, and you will develop a tolerance to it with high daily use. You will need more and more to get that hit from it you want. Once overstimulating becomes the norm, you think you are performing at your best, but you're not. You are always going to be a couple of steps behind it, a wired shadow of yourself, because you are using caffeine simply to get to the point at which you *can* perform.

Studies show caffeine is at its most beneficial in athletes at moderate quantities of around 3–6 milligrams per kilogram of body mass (that's about 6–13 milligrams per pound),[4] and the Food and Drug Administration recommends 400 milligrams as the daily maximum intake of caffeine for the average person. To put that in perspective, a Starbucks grande brewed coffee contains 330 milligrams. The same chain's single espresso contains 75 milligrams, and a home-brewed cup of coffee can contain as much as 200 milligrams.

On top of this, caffeine has a half-life of up to six hours, which means it will be present in your body much longer than you might think. Deciding not to drink caffeine later in the day to aid your nocturnal sleep is all well and good, but what if you've already had a Starbucks grande, a coffee from the machine at work, a couple of cups of tea (each of which could contain anywhere from 25 to 100 milligrams), and a can of Coke (35 milligrams) with your lunch? And then there are the things we consume that we might not be aware contain caffeine, such as chocolate, certain painkillers, and even decaffeinated tea and coffee (decaffeinated definitely doesn't mean the same as caffeine-free).

If you are overstimulating on caffeine in an unregimented way, day after day, you aren't using it like we use it in sports. You are using it habitually, rather than for a specific event. No one is suggesting you can't have that great cup of coffee you crave—the legions of Lycra-clad cyclists sipping espresso outside cafés all over the country here in the United Kingdom are testament to that—but why not get a measure on how much you are consuming, and use it strategically? If you have a meeting you need to be sharp for, or a piece of work that requires the very best of your concentration and focus, why not save it for this? Use caffeine as a performance enhancer, instead of simply to get yourself to a position from which you can perform.

Managing Your Chronotype

Daylight is a more effective tool in the long term than an out-of-control caffeine habit. For the PMer, daylight in the morning is vital if you want to set your body clock to play catch-up with the AMers. Get a dawn simulator, which recreates a sunrise in your bedroom to wake you up, from a reputable brand such as Lumie or Philips; open the curtains, go outside.

The really bad news for PMers is that you should stop sleeping in on the weekend too. If you spend all week adjusting your body clock to the demands of your job and then let it all go on the weekend, your clock will drift back toward its natural, slower state, and you'll be starting over come Monday. The symptoms of your social jet lag will be so much worse.

Offices and workplaces should take this more seriously. Instead of having hierarchies where the more senior people get offices with a window, allocate them to the PMers when they're struggling through their morning and to the AMers for their afternoon. Investing in daylight lamps will help both the AMers and PMers conquer their respective difficult parts of the day and increase their productivity, especially in winter, when there is less light. For the soccer teams I work with, I put daylight lamps in the locker rooms. The players don't notice—they're just lamps to them—and you could do the same thing in meeting rooms.

It's not all bad news for PMers. They have a natural advantage not only when it comes to enjoying nightlife but also when working nighttime shifts. An AMer nurse working night shifts in a hospital would equally be in need of daylight lamps and caffeine to play catch-up with PMer colleagues. The most important thing for either chronotype to find is some harmony with their environment.

If we go back to our fire on the island and assume that you're a PMer and I'm an AMer, as we return to the natural rhythms of our respective body clocks, we'd learn to start working in harmony. You would sit up and keep watch, tending the fire and taking on camp chores for the evening, while I drifted off to sleep, and then in the morning, when I woke an hour or two before you, I would get the fire started again, cook us breakfast, and prepare for the day ahead.

Back in the real world, we can use this to benefit our daily lives. An AMer might live with his partner, a PMer, and they both have to leave for work at 8:30 a.m. He gets up at 6:30 and she gets up at 8, but, of course, every time he gets up in the morning, he disturbs his partner. She goes back to sleep and imagines it's doing her good, but in reality she's flitting between wakefulness and sleep. But what if a compromise could be made? They both get up at 7 instead, which is a big shift for her, but the AMer makes the breakfast and gives the PMer the space to sit in daylight, to reset her body clock and wake up naturally. It will take a bit of adjusting to, but all of a sudden the couple are working more in harmony. When the evening comes around, it is the PMer's turn to do her part, maybe cooking dinner or doing the dishes later, when the AMer is tired.

If you're an AMer, you know you're at your best in the morning, so you can plan your day to take advantage of this. Let's say your job involves managing your company's social media accounts, some bookkeeping, and a lot of communication, but also some of the more mundane realities of office life such as taking the mail to the post office and filing. Presuming you have a bit of freedom in the order in which you do things, you could manipulate your schedule so that you compose all your tweets and press releases in the morning, everything that requires you to be at your most alert, and then spend your afternoon doing the mailing and filing. Speaking as an AMer myself, if you want to give me some accounts that need to be added up correctly, I'd advise you to ask me in the morning.

Often there isn't this kind of freedom in our daily work, and sometimes a job that involves writing a press release or something that similarly requires thought will land on your desk in the afternoon and it has to be done right at that moment. But where we're able to, instead of spending what feels like forever on getting something done in the afternoon, wondering why it's taking so long, just stop and think about it. If you're struggling with it now, come back to it in the morning, when you're fresher and more alert. It's the same philosophy with PMers.

I will identify the chronotype of each player on a team I'm working with, which is of benefit to both the performers and their coaches. Player B, mentioned at the start of the chapter, is a PMer, while Player A is an AMer, but their coach didn't know that. However, if I've been brought in to work with the team and I identify this and talk to Player B, it becomes clear to him why he's struggling to get out of bed first thing, why he needs that alarm, and why he's not so great at practices in the morning. I can give him some advice on what he can do about it.

From the coach's point of view, he now knows that it might not just be a case of bad discipline, because Player B's makeup means he naturally doesn't want to practice in the morning—he'd prefer to do it in the afternoon. The manager's not about to split practices and tell the AMers and PMers to come in separately, of course, but he now knows that he needs to make some adjustments. He can't keep making Player B do everything in the morning because something eventually will give. He might not manage to shake that lingering injury fully, or he might just do something silly in the heat of the moment in a big game, because the coach has been pushing him in a manner that goes against his biological makeup.

It also gives the coach a little more insight late on a spring evening during the NBA Finals with the series on the line. Player A is an AMer. He's masking it, playing late into the night, but the choice between him and the similarly skilled Player B is no choice at all, really: the PMer is more alert and he's in his element in the evening. He should take to the court, where he'd stand a better chance of making that crucial last-second shot.

CHRONOTYPE:
SEVEN STEPS TO SLEEP SMARTER

1. Know your chronotype, and establish those of close friends and family. Use the University of Munich questionnaire if you're not sure.

2. Manipulate your day so you can be at your best when it matters most.

3. Use caffeine as a strategic performance enhancer, not out of habit—and no more than 400 milligrams per day.

4. PMers, sleep in on weekends if you want to beat social jet lag.

5. Equip meeting rooms, offices, and desks with daylight lamps to improve alertness, productivity, and mood at work.

6. Know when to put yourself forward and when to take a backseat. Should you step up in a late-night game when you're an AMer?

7. Learn to work in harmony with your partner if your chronotypes differ.

THREE

A Game of Ninety Minutes

Sleeping in Cycles, Not Hours

You wake up to darkness. *How long have I been asleep?* you wonder. After getting up and going to the bathroom, you check your
phone: 3:07. That's OK—plenty of time left in bed. If you get
back to sleep now, you're still on course for around eight hours
when your alarm goes off at 7:30. You've got a big day tomorrow, lots to do at work. You need to be fresh. You need your
eight hours.

So you lie there for a while. And then a while longer. You
check your phone: 3:33. That's still OK. Plenty of time. You have
that big 10 a.m. meeting, of course, so you have to be fresh.
And how is that going to go? you ask yourself, and the butterflies
begin again; your shoulders, almost imperceptibly, have tight-
ened. You're no longer lying on your side; you've switched to
your back, fingers interlinked behind your head. *All the better
for thinking.* You check the time once more: 3:56. Something
about the proximity to 4 a.m., about losing a whole hour before

23

tomorrow, of all days, fills you with a dread unique to these hours of the night.

The taunting numerals 5:53 are the last thing you remember before your alarm shocks you from sleep at 7:30, with your mouth parched and a growing ache behind your eyes. You haven't had anywhere near eight hours. How are you going to manage today?

One Size Fits All?

If you were asked to think of a number, any number, between one and ten, given that you're reading a book about sleep, it's likely you'll think eight. Eight hours of sleep each night is a nice round number, but it is one of the enduring pieces of so-called sleep wisdom that doesn't add up for everyone.

The idea of eight hours a night is a relatively modern one. We'll talk about sleeping in more than one phase later in the book, but for now it's enough to say that until the nineteenth century, with the industrial revolution and the introduction of artificial light, it is unlikely that people were sleeping in a single eight-hour chunk at nighttime. It's unlikelier still that they were worrying about it.

Eight hours is the *average* amount of sleep people get per night, and it somehow seems to have become a recommended amount—for everyone. The resultant pressure people put on getting this is incredibly damaging and counterproductive to getting the right amount we individually need.

This one-size-fits-all mentality doesn't apply to other areas of our lives. With things like calorie consumption, there is an industry-accepted standard in differences for the sexes, and that's before we consider the difference in need between a Herculean fitness fanatic and someone who lives a largely sedentary lifestyle. There are guidelines for maximum daily consumption of things like sugar and salt, but having less than these amounts is considered acceptable. There is no definitive length of time that should be spent on daily exercise (more than the recommended amount is usually good). It is only in sleep—and, as we'll learn later, not only in this aspect of sleep—that such wisdom is simply accepted.

The truth is that each of us is different. There are the Margaret Thatchers and Marissa Mayers of this world, getting by on four to six hours each night while running Britain or being CEO of Yahoo, respectively, and then there are people like tennis legend Roger Federer and fastest-man-ever Usain Bolt, who say they need as much as ten hours per night.

And even allowing for these extremes, our need for sleep changes throughout our lives. As children and then adolescents, we need much more sleep than we do as adults. According to the National Sleep Foundation, the average teenager (fourteen to seventeen years old) needs between eight and ten hours of sleep. The average adult needs between seven and nine.

If you need less than eight hours of sleep per night but you're forcing yourself to try to get eight, going to bed when you're not tired and lying there awake, you're wasting your time. If you're looking at the clock in the middle of the night, anxiously calculating how much short of eight hours you're going to be, tossing, turning, and growing more and more concerned about getting *enough* sleep, you're doing likewise—you're wasting your valuable time on not sleeping.

Shift workers, airline staff, financial traders, long-distance truck drivers—they're not getting eight hours per night. The athletes I work with don't get eight hours per night, and that's not only because of the pressures on their time. It's because they don't look at sleeping in hours; they do it in cycles.

The Cycles of Sleep

The R90 approach simply means *recovery in 90 minutes*. I haven't randomly picked a number, any number, between one and a hundred; ninety minutes is the length of time it takes a person under clinical conditions to go through the stages of sleep that constitute a cycle.

Our sleep cycles are composed of four (or sometimes five) distinct stages, and it's easy to think about our passage through a cycle as being like a journey down a flight of stairs. When we turn the lights off and get into bed at night, we're at the top of the stairs. Down at the bottom of the stairs is deep sleep, which is where we want to get to.

The Top of the Stairs: Dozing Off
Non-REM (NREM) Stage 1

We're slowly taking our first couple of steps down the staircase, and we're somewhere between awake and asleep for a few minutes. Have you ever jerked awake suddenly because you feel like you're falling? That happens in this stage and it's just a hallucination, but it means we need to begin our descent down the stairs again. It's very easy to pull us back up the stairs from here—a door opening or a voice in the street outside will do it—but once we manage to negotiate this stage successfully, we make our way down to . . .

The Middle of the Stairs: Light Sleep
NREM Stage 2

In light sleep our heart rate slows and our body temperature drops. From here, we can still be dragged back to the top of the stairs by hearing someone shouting our name or, in the case of a mother (and women are biologically susceptible to this), her baby crying. We spend the biggest percentage of our time asleep in this state, so it can feel like a long flight of stairs at times, particularly for those getting stuck in light sleep, but it isn't time wasted if it's part of a well-balanced cycle. Information consolidation and improved motor skill performance are linked to this stage.[1] And as we move further down, we begin the transition to the really good stuff.

The Bottom of the Stairs: Deep Sleep
NREM Stage 3 (and 4)

Congratulations—you've reached the bottom of the stairs. Down here, it takes a good deal of effort to wake us. If you've ever had to shake someone awake, or if you've been unfortunate enough to be on the receiving end and woken up feeling punch-drunk and confused, you'll understand the kind of power deep sleep has and the effects of sleep inertia. For the sleepwalkers among us, this is the stage when you will take to the floor.

Our brain produces delta waves, the slowest-frequency brainwaves, in deep sleep (we produce the high-frequency beta waves when we are awake). We want to spend as much time as we can down here, wallowing in it, as this is where we reap the major physically restorative benefits of sleep, such as the increase in our release of growth hormone.[2] Human growth hormone (HGH) might be familiar to some readers as a banned performance-enhancing drug in sports, but our bodies produce it naturally, and its effects are powerful. Dr. Michael J. Breus, a clinical psychologist and sleep expert, describes it as "a key in-gredient we all need routinely to grow new cells, repair tissues, recover our bodies from the daily grinds, and essentially be (and feel) rejuvenated." We hope to spend around 20 percent of our time down here in deep sleep during the night.

Helter Skelter: REM

In the song "Helter Skelter," the Beatles sing about going back up to the top of the slide, where they stop and turn, then go for a ride. It's not too dissimilar to this stage of sleep. We head back up the stairs, to light-sleep territory for a while, before we reach a stage of sleep many of us are familiar with: REM (rapid eye movement). This is where our mind takes us on a ride—we do most of our dreaming in this stage while our bodies are tempo-rarily paralyzed, and REM sleep is believed to have beneficial ef-fects on creativity.[3] We need to get back up toward the top, stop and turn, and go for a ride every bit as much as we need to get to the bottom of the stairs. And again, we should be looking to spend around 20 percent of our time in this stage. Infants spend more like half their time asleep here. At the end of the REM stage we wake up—we usually won't remember this—before be-ginning the next cycle.

Each cycle during the night is different. Deep sleep accounts for a higher portion of our sleep in earlier cycles, as our body prioritizes getting this as soon as it can, while REM sleep accounts for a higher portion in later cycles. *However*, if we have been getting less sleep than normal, our brain will drop into REM for longer in earlier cycles, demonstrating its importance to us.[4] This is just one of the reasons why trying to "catch up" on sleep—by going to bed earlier than normal or sleeping in later—is a waste of your time. Once sleep has been lost, it's gone. But our bodies are remarkably good at doing our catching up for us.

Ideally, we would spend a night in bed smoothly making the transition from one cycle to the next, in a pattern of sleep-wake-sleep-wake, gradually getting less deep sleep and more REM sleep as the night progresses, until our final wake-up in the morning. This is the key to getting the right *quality* of sleep: all the light sleep, deep sleep, and REM we need in a series of cycles that feels to us like one long continuous night's sleep.

However, there are all sorts of obstacles in our way. Noise, age, stress, medication, caffeine, physical disturbances like a partner's leg touching us, breathing through our mouths instead of our noses, snoring and sleep apnea, temperature, and the necessity of a bathroom visit can bring us back up toward the top of the stairs and leave some of us doomed to spend too much of the night in the lighter stages of sleep, or take us out of our cycles entirely.

The repercussions can range from growing levels of daytime fatigue to far more serious incidents. Our bodies can dump us straight down into a micro-sleep during the day when we least expect it, such as when driving a car or operating a piece of machinery.

If we're trapped in light-sleeping patterns, then it doesn't matter how much sleep we're getting—we're not benefiting from it fully. The R90 approach tackles the obstacles that stop us from getting down the stairs, and it all starts with our morning alarm.

Wake Up!

Flexibility seems like a desirable trait in the modern world. Late nights, weekends, and travel mean that it should pay to avoid fixed approaches to life. If you had a couple of drinks and some food after work, doesn't it make sense to set the alarm a bit later for the next morning to give yourself a bit more sleep? And surely it's best to forget about the alarm altogether on a day off, isn't it?

In fact, setting a constant wake time is one of the most powerful tools at our disposal when looking to improve the quality of our recovery. Our bodies love it when our circadian rhythms, set by the rise and fall of the sun, work around a consistent point, and our minds love it because this constant wake time can help us build the confidence to be more flexible in other aspects of our lives.

Picking a constant wake time requires a little thought, and more than a little effort, because you should *get up* at this time too. It's advisable to look back over the previous two or three months of your life, factoring in your work and personal life, and choose the earliest time you have to get up. The time should be one that is achievable every day and there should be nothing in your life that requires you to be up earlier except for special circumstances, such as an early flight. So don't pick 7:30 a.m. if you occasionally have to be up at 7 a.m. to get to a meeting. You pick 7 a.m. in that instance. And remember, you will be using this wake time on the weekend too, so don't choose something completely unrealistic on the assumption that you can sleep later on your days off.

Give some thought to your chronotype. If you're a PMer, don't pick something far earlier than when you have to get up, but do bear in mind that it should have some relation to when the sun comes up. The further you get from that, the more you depart from the circadian process. For a PMer who has to be up for work at a time that is at odds with their natural rhythms, this wake time is going to be essential for resetting their clock every day so that they can keep up with the AMers and in-betweeners.

Once you've established the earliest time you need to be up, make that your wake time. Ideally, your wake time should be at least ninety minutes before you have to be at work or class or any other obligation, so that you can have enough time to prepare yourself after sleep.

You will need an alarm to wake you, especially to start with, but what you will find is that your body and mind become trained to get up at this time. Before long you'll find yourself turning off the alarm before it sounds because you're already awake.

Using your wake time, you can now count backward in ninety-minute cycles to establish when you should aim to be asleep. If you're the average person, aiming to get around eight hours in at night, that would be the equivalent of five cycles per night (which equates to seven and a half hours). If you've chosen 7:30 a.m. as your wake time, then you should be aiming to be asleep by midnight, which means curling up and letting go fifteen minutes before—or however long it takes you to get off to sleep.

When I start working with an athlete and I ask them how long they slept the night before, they're likely to give a vague answer. "Oh, about seven or eight hours," they might say. But athletes, just like the rest of us, have a random approach to it. They *think* they went to bed around eleven, they're pretty sure they woke up to go to the bathroom once during the night, and, as far as they remember, it was around 7 or 7:30 a.m. when they got up. The night before, who knows?

Setting a constant wake time eliminates the random nature of our sleep. It helps us instill a routine that gives us the confidence to know how much we're getting. If I ask the same question of an athlete I've been working with for a while, they will answer without hesitation: "I got five cycles in last night."

Do that every night and you've got a thirty-five-cycle week, which is simply perfection. It's also never going to happen. Life gets in the way: a night game for a football player, or a delayed train home, a late dinner, a book we can't put down, or a phone call from an old friend for the rest of us. You need to have the flexibility to work with this, to still enjoy your life and get by at work without worrying about bedtime. So this isn't fixed. You get up at exactly the same time every day, but you have ninety-minute intervals in which to go to bed—although you should not use the one before your ideal bedtime. As we've said previously, there's no catching up on lost sleep.

So if you get home a bit later and you're not prepared to go naturally into a sleep state at midnight for your chosen wake

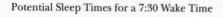

Potential Sleep Times for a 7:30 Wake Time

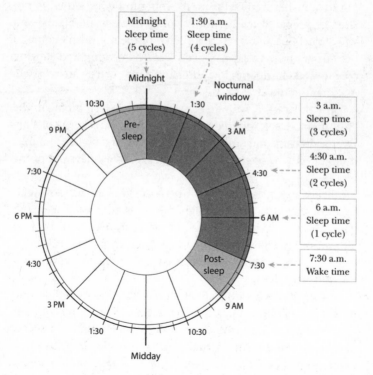

time of 7:30 a.m., you can go to sleep at 1:30 a.m., which is four cycles (six hours); come in even later and you can go to bed at 3 a.m., only three cycles. Now you're pushing it. Now you're working at the margins, like the athletes I work with. They love the idea of these ninety-minute slots: they're measurable and achievable. Soccer players like them because they're the same length as a match. They know that when an event demands it, they can start manipulating these cycles for their own purposes. They are in control of their recovery, rather than the other way around.

Scheduling Sleep

Worrying about sleep is an obstacle many of us face when trying to get what we need from it. Going to bed when we're not tired or prepared for it is only going to cause problems, and stressing about waking in the middle of the night isn't going to help us get back to sleep. Once we start worrying and stewing over it, stress hormones like adrenaline and cortisol are released, making us more alert.

For those of us who don't suffer from a sleep problem, the "bad night's sleep" often occurs in isolation, or as a part of a period of pressure and stress. If taken as part of a broader sample, it might only be one day out of a week, or a few days out of the month.

I talk about sleep in cycles per week, not hours per night. So all of a sudden, one bad night out of seven doesn't seem too bad. We immediately take the pressure off, because it isn't an all-or-nothing eight hours per night. Everything isn't riding on tonight. Instead, someone who needs five cycles a night is aiming for thirty-five per week.

I will sit down with a client and look at their schedule, and I'll show them how they can achieve this. We will look at their week ahead and flag where the problem areas are. For a soccer player we would identify things like a Thursday evening away game as an issue. The game won't end until well into the night, and there may be post-game interviews afterward, adrenaline to come down from, and travel to take into account. The player isn't going to get their five cycles in that night. So we'll look at how they can compensate for them.

We try to avoid three consecutive nights of fewer than five cycles. Instead, we'd look to follow a night or two of this with the ideal routine. If we can get at least four nights in a week of an ideal routine in our schedules, then we're doing OK. Most important, we're aware of how much sleep we're getting. We can see quite clearly if we're pushing things too much. Five nights of fewer cycles in a week when it's not part of a short-term regimen change? We need to look at that.

"Give a man a fish and you feed him for a day; teach a man to fish and you feed him for a lifetime," says the proverb, and it applies just the same to the R90 program. I'll reach a point with a client when I can hand their schedules to them and say, "I know you can get thirty cycles out of this. Whether you do is up to you." It's all in their hands from then on.

It is empowering for anyone to take control of their sleep like this, and it is possible to start manipulating cycles in the short term to free up more time for a specific event or period in our lives as part of a controlled regimen change. An athlete gearing up for the Olympic Games might switch from a five-cycle routine to four cycles per night, which frees up almost two extra days per month. There is confidence to be gained in knowing that time can be unlocked, even if it's only temporarily. Some people switch from five cycles to four and find that they function better. They're not waking up during the night anymore. They know how much sleep they need now. They feel refreshed and optimistic that there are enough hours in the day after all.

You can do this in your own life. Start on five cycles, and see how you feel after seven days. If this is too long, move it down to four. Not enough? Move up to six. You'll know because you should feel good once you've adjusted to it. What I really want is for you to feel the confidence that you are in control of your sleep. Once you're comfortable with what you think is your ideal night, then you can look at adjusting it to fit with the demands of your lifestyle. Just like an elite athlete, you should look to follow two nights of fewer cycles with your ideal one, and achieve at least four ideal routines per week.

There's no need to panic if you're not always adhering to this—just like there's no need for all that witching-hour worry about getting eight hours that night—because you are starting to take charge of your sleep. Through scheduling it, you are able to see where you are getting less and where problems may be occurring, instead of simply feeling you haven't slept enough without having any kind of evidence to back it up with and identify where you can make changes to your routine.

Once you're comfortable with sleeping in cycles, you can start to emulate the Olympians preparing for the Games in making short-term regimen changes for a specific set of circumstances. If you are training for a marathon and you have to fit in your training around your job, you can cut down on your cycles at night to make it work. If you are involved in a project that is making more demands on your life, move down to a four-cycle routine to get it done. If you're really being pushed in the short term, see if you can get down to three.

You might now be saying to yourself, *Wait a minute—I can't manage on three or four cycles per night!* But that's because you're still thinking about sleeping in a monophasic way, purely as one block each night, instead of as a twenty-four-hour recovery process with the other windows and opportunities this offers us to compensate for fewer cycles at night. And you're not yet seeing the time we spend preparing to go to bed and how we spend it after we have slept as a non-negotiable component of this. As you will see in the next two chapters, sleep is about so much more than the time spent doing it at night.

CYCLES, NOT HOURS: SEVEN STEPS TO SLEEP SMARTER

1. Your constant wake time is the anchor that holds in place the R90 technique. Set one and stick to it. If you share your bed with a partner, get that person to do the same, and ideally make them the same time.

2. Think of sleep in ninety-minute cycles, not hours.

3. Your sleep time is flexible, but it is determined by counting back in ninety-minute slots from your wake time.

4. Look at sleep in a broader tract of time to take the pressure off. One "bad night's sleep" won't kill you—think of it in terms of cycles per week.

5. Try to avoid three back-to-back nights of fewer cycles than your ideal.

6. It's not simply quality vs. quantity. Know how much you need. For the average person, thirty-five cycles per week is ideal. Twenty-eight (six hours per night) to thirty is OK. If you're getting anything less that isn't planned for, you might be overdoing it.

7. Aim to achieve your ideal amount at least four times per week.

FOUR

Warming Up and Cooling Down

Pre- and Post-Sleep Routines

It's been a long day. You arrive home somewhere close to 11 p.m. after staying a few extra hours at the office to work and then joining a couple of colleagues for a late dinner and a few glasses of wine. You kick off your shoes, undress, and throw your clothes in a crumpled pile on the floor before brushing your teeth in the unforgiving glow of the bathroom light. Finally you head to the bedroom and get under the covers next to your partner, who wakes up briefly, then turns over and goes back to sleep. You're full and tired, and you have been looking forward to this all the way home in the taxi. You close your eyes and drift away . . .

You jerk awake suddenly, your mind racing with the conversation at dinner. What did your colleagues mean by some of the things that were said? Did you come across a little unprofessional—maybe even a little rude—in what you said about others in the office?

Now you're awake. Your mind is moving on to other matters: Will you be able to finish your current project on time? Are you going to be late again with it? How will that look?

Your heart is speeding up, and your old friend indigestion has arrived after the dinner you finished just an hour ago. You're twitchy and uncomfortable. Should you get up or stick it out in bed? You're absolutely beat—why on earth can't you just go off to sleep?

The Before and After

If I arrived home sometime around 11 p.m.—my ideal sleep time to get five cycles in before my constant wake time of 6:30 a.m.—I would not come in, brush my teeth, and jump straight into bed. Instead, I would wait for the next slot, at 12:30 a.m., and I would be in for a four-cycle night. How else would I fit my pre-sleep routine in?

"Fail to prepare, prepare to fail" is a phrase that could have been written with pre- and post-sleep recovery in mind. What you do immediately before you go to bed has a direct effect on the quality and duration of your sleep, while what you do after waking has significant consequences for the rest of your day (and the coming night).

In the R90 program, we look at these pre- and post-sleep periods as being just as important as the time spent actually asleep. In fact, they're more important, because you can exercise some direct control over them. It is here that we start looking at ninety minutes not just as segments of the time you spend asleep, but as portions of your waking day. Ideally, you would have a ninety-minute period for pre-sleep and the same amount for post-sleep.

Looking at it like this, a four-cycle routine is not only six hours of sleep at night but also nine hours dedicated to the process of rest and recovery. That isn't to say you need to block off ninety minutes every morning and night when you do nothing but prepare for sleep or for the day ahead. It's more about toning down what you are doing, setting aside the unhelpful factors that will inhibit the hours you're about to spend either sleeping or dealing with the challenges of your waking day, and introducing aspects that better fit your circadian rhythms and chronotype.

Pre-Sleep

Your pre-sleep routine is the preparation to make sure you are in a state ready to go to sleep. It's the work you do to put yourself in a position where you can start your first cycle and then move seamlessly through the subsequent cycles during the night, getting as much of the light and deep sleep and REM as you need.

Much like a Team Sky cyclist would with their marginal gains when approaching an event, when we're heading toward going into a sleep state, a position in which we're vulnerable for several hours, we need to start pushing aside the things that are going to get in the way of this.

If you've eaten late, then you need to set aside this factor by not going straight to bed. Being full and digesting food is going to interfere with your circadian urge to suppress the bowel at around 9 or 10 p.m., and it's going to affect the quality of your sleep. Alcohol, despite having the capability to give us a pleasantly drowsy feeling, affects the quality of sleep when consumed to excess. If you've had several fraught work conversations, then you're not going to just stop thinking about them as soon as you jump into bed. You need to download your thoughts. You need your pre-sleep routine.

On an ordinary night at home, when I'm planning to be asleep by 11 p.m., I will start preparing for it at 9:30. Nothing dramatic happens—I don't bolt out of my chair and cry out, "Let's ready the pre-sleep!" But I know that if I'm still a little hungry, I need to have a light snack; I need to take in my last fluids for the night, so that I don't wake up thirsty. And I will empty my bladder, because I don't want to be woken with the urge to go to the bathroom during the night.

Pre-sleep isn't just about addressing the seemingly obvious bodily functions before bed. There is a multitude of other factors that we can work with to ensure that we're fully prepared to enter a sleep state.

Technology Shutdown

Putting a stop to computers, tablets, smartphones, and televisions in the period before sleep will restrict your exposure to the artificial light these devices emit. For those who can't live without their tech before bedtime, software such as f.lux and Apple's Night Shift mode on its mobile operating systems will "warm" the color temperature on devices, reducing the amount of blue light. But this doesn't solve the other problem with tech before bedtime: its effect on our stress levels and capacity to keep our brains alert.

If you're responding to emails and messages right up until bedtime, you're keeping yourself open to potentially stressful situations. The message you receive fifteen minutes before you go to bed could be the kind that will keep your mind whirring when you're trying to sleep. You might struggle to get to sleep before you receive a reply to the message *you've* sent—something even more out of your control to worry about.

If we put a curfew on our emails and messages, we can deal with any potentially stressful situations at least ninety minutes before bed. If you're the type to get stressed while waiting for a reply to a message you've just sent, then you could draft your message and hold off on sending it until the morning—which is a bit like sticking a stamp on a letter to get it ready to mail. This way you're taking control not only of your correspondence but also of your availability. You're saying that you're not always on hand to answer 10 p.m. emails.

Personal messages are, of course, slightly different. If you're in the throes of a new relationship, you're not going to stay away from your phone for an hour and a half before bed if there's a chance of receiving a text message from your lover. Who knows what you might be missing out on? But simply reducing *any* of your tech usage in this period before sleep—shutting down laptops, tablets, and similar devices, putting a stop to work email, saying no to a high-octane action movie or video game in bed on your flat-screen television with high-definition sound—would be a good start.

Some people are already very good at this. I see an increasing number of email signatures and out-of-office replies saying "I only check email three times a day" or making clear that they are not connected 24/7 to their email. For them, it's easy to shut down the tech. But for the rest of us, it's not enough to simply take a prescriptive approach and say, "Don't do this." How do you stop it if you don't know how?

One great step is to identify how often you check your device throughout the day and for what reason (texts, email, alerts, and social media, both work-related and non-work-related). Apple revealed that the average iPhone user unlocks their phone eighty times a day, which sounds like a lot until you start monitoring how often you do it. For most of us, it's at least every time we receive an alert.

If we look at finding a window during the day when we can have a break from technology and do something pleasurable instead, we can start to take control of it. If you leave your phone behind when you exercise—swimming is a particularly good option, as even the most tech-addicted person doesn't want to get their smartphone wet, but it could just as easily be heading to the gym or going for a walk—you are creating a reward for your body and mind in the form of the benefits of the exercise and allowing them to be free of the need to constantly respond to alerts and messages.

It doesn't just have to be exercise. You could put the phone away on your journey to work and read a book instead, or you could leave your phone locked in your drawer when you go for lunch with a friend or colleague—all of which gives your brain that association between pleasure and a technology break.

Once you're comfortable doing this, you'll be better able to integrate it into your pre-sleep routine (which is itself a reward for your body and mind) and ensure that your phone goes to sleep when you do.

There are, of course, some helpful applications tech can provide us with during this period. There are many mindfulness and meditation apps that can be used to relax us as we prepare to sleep, and if they work for you, stick with them (though the device they are used on should ideally be kept out of the bedroom or removed after use, if possible).

From Warm to Cool

When we were out on our island in Chapter 1, the temperature dropped when the sun set and we started to become ready for sleep. Our body temperature naturally drops in the evening, as part of our circadian rhythms, but things like central heating can interfere with it. We can overcome this and tap into our biological urge at home through a couple of shortcuts.

First, while it might seem obvious, make sure your comforter or blanket isn't too warm or too cold. It might make sense to you to curl up in a toasty bed, but once your body temperature gets to work with it, you will start to overheat and possibly perspire heavily, all of which can pull you out of a sleep cycle. Hanging your leg out from the covers, which requires conscious thought, may work for a bit, but ultimately disturbed and broken sleep will prevail. Hot-water bottles and electric blankets are a no-no, unless you're using them to reduce the bite in a particularly cold room or you are especially sensitive to temperature.

Keeping the bedroom itself cool (not cold) is important. In winter you could do this by turning off the radiator or turning down the thermostat in the bedroom when you're trying to enter sleep. You could have a warm (not hot) rinse under the shower, just to raise your body temperature a degree or two, so that when you get into your cooler bed, you're approximating that shift in temperature from day to night.

In summer, keeping the curtains or blinds closed all day and ventilating the room can help keep it a degree or two cooler than the rest of the home. Sleeping with just a sheet or the duvet cover (with the comforter itself removed) will help. For those of us who have air-conditioning, use this to cool the room prior to sleeping on a particularly hot night; those who don't have it could use a fan with a bottle of frozen water placed in front of it.

Some people find having a shower before bed is a helpful part of their pre-sleep because they feel more comfortable getting into bed clean, but you don't need to have a full shower; just a quick rinse will do. Like much of the advice in this chapter, it's about finding what works for you.

From Light to Dark

Our body clocks respond to the shift from light to dark. We start producing melatonin so that we will become sleepy, but many of the things we surround ourselves with as bedtime approaches interfere with this. We've already mentioned our technology, but there are several other areas in which we could look to improve.

Dimming everything down as you enter your pre-sleep is a good idea. Turn the main lights in your home off, and have less-powerful lamps with warm-color bulbs—red or amber, which will not affect you in the same way blue light does—or candles in your living room and bedroom to provide ambient lighting. Of course, it's easy to undo all this good work by then brushing your teeth before bed in the blazing fluorescent light of the bathroom. One solution would be to brush your teeth earlier, and another would be to change the bulb in the bathroom to something less dazzling. Or what about a candle? If you have gotten into the habit of standing in front of the mirror next to your partner while you both brush your teeth in silence under the unforgiving glare of the bathroom light, night after night, doing it instead in the light from a candle might make for a welcome break from this recurring pre-sleep nightmare. It's hardly a candlelit dinner as far as romance is concerned, but it lends an extra element of occasion to a very mundane part of your pre-sleep routine, and it might just help you sleep a little easier.

You should be able to put your sleeping environment in darkness or blackout so as to replicate the circadian process. Most of us will have some kind of artificial light intruding into our bedrooms, especially if we live in a town or city. So make sure the curtains or blinds are sufficient to keep the light out. That means no little gaps around the curtains where the light can creep in. Invest in some blackout blinds if necessary. On the Grand Tours in the glamorous world of professional cycling, I will sometimes tape black trash bags over the riders' hotel room windows to keep the light out.

If you like to read before you go to sleep, consider doing it outside the bedroom, so that you're moving from light (in the room where you're reading) to the dark of your bedroom. If reading in bed is a pre-sleep ritual and you'd rather toss and turn all night than go without it, then consider turning off your lamp when you've finished reading, leaving the room, and coming back into the dark room before going to bed. Dawn simulators have a setting to go gradually from light to dark, which you could use too.

Everything in Its Right Place

With the emphasis of your pre-sleep routine being on moving away from using televisions, smartphones, and laptops, it's possible you might be wondering, *What's left for me to do?*

This is a good time to declutter. I'm not talking about emptying your house out as part of a fashionable lifestyle craze, but rather about taking some positive actions in your environment so that once you're either asleep or preparing to go to sleep, your mind can be free of little niggling thoughts about packing your bag in the morning, remembering to take your dry cleaning with you to work, or the sudden realization that you're out of tea bags. It's incredible what can pop into our minds at night.

Doing some simple, non-stimulating tasks around the home to better prepare you for the next day will take care of this and give your mind the space it needs. This might involve ironing and hanging up your clothes, tidying your environment, taking out the recycling, and putting everything in place for the morning. Don't worry if you're not the obsessively tidy type—it can equally involve throwing your clothes on the chair where they belong and dumping your bag on the floor by the front door so you don't forget it. Everything in the right (for you) place.

Rather than leave the dishes for the morning, now would be a good time to do them. It's a simple task, not requiring much effort or energy, and it means you go to bed with the kitchen clean. Whether you're aware of it or not, it's one less thing for you to have on your mind during the night. If you normally put the dishwasher or washing machine on at night, for convenience or because electricity is cheaper, stop and think about this. You might not hear it when you first go to bed, but what about if you wake up during the night? Do you hear it then, when the world is much quieter and new noises become audible? Put it on at a different time if it isn't far away enough not to have an impact.

Using this period of time to get your little essentials right for the next day will declutter your mind for the night ahead. And when the little everyday thoughts are taken care of, it leaves you time to take care of the bigger problems.

Downloading Your Day

One of the strongest pulls to take you out of a sleep cycle is thought: ruminating about the day you've just experienced, worrying about the one ahead. According to the American Psychological Association, some 43 percent of American adults reported that stress had caused them to lie awake at night at least once during the previous month.[1] Reducing unhelpful tech in the lead-up to bedtime helps prevent any fresh anxieties entering the equation, but it won't eliminate existing troubles.

There are millions of tiny moments that accumulate and make up each of our days—a conversation with a colleague, the commute, lunch with a friend, using a new piece of software at work, daydreaming while looking out of the window—and the brain must digest them. Indeed, scientists believe one of the key reasons we sleep is to process our experiences into memories and consolidate learned skills.[2]

We can better prepare our minds for this by downloading our day. We take all of our experiences over the course of the day and file them away, ready for our mind to digest them as we sleep. The simple tasks just described help us do this, and there are other methods to incorporate in our pre-sleep routines that can do it too. Some people find meditating and breathing exercises useful, and if this is something that helps you download your day, then you should make it part of your routine.

I find it helpful to take a piece of paper and a pencil and simply write a "what's on my mind" list, addressing any thoughts I have and anything that has worried or concerned me during that day. It's not my actual to-do list, which is safely saved on my calendar in the cloud, but something more personal. If a particular piece of business has been on my mind, I might write down a note to call the client in the morning; if a birthday of a loved one or something like Mother's Day is on the horizon, I could draw a bunch of flowers as a reminder. I'm just scribbling on the page, even doodling at times, in a very relaxed, informal process that can be done at any spare moment before going to bed. I will then leave that piece of paper next to my house keys—or anything I never leave home without—for the next morning, so I won't forget it.

Putting it all down on paper means that I go to bed feeling that I have consciously addressed the issue for now, and I can trust the work that goes on in my sleeping brain to take care of it overnight.

Security

Going into a sleep state is the most vulnerable position we will put ourselves in all day, so we need to feel as secure as possible. Locking all the doors and windows, or double-checking that they're all locked, will help instill this feeling of safety. And, like the downloading of our day, it will eliminate the unhelpful thoughts—such as *Did I leave the bathroom window open?*—that will prevent us from entering a sleep state.

Sleep Exercise

Strenuous exercise should be avoided in the period prior to sleep (unless it's sex, of course, which we'll talk about later in the book). It elevates your heart rate, body temperature, and adrenaline, and the glaring light and pounding music in many gyms are about as far from the two of us sitting by the fire as is possible. But a bit of light exercise—a short walk around the block before bedtime, some yoga such as sun salutations, a gentle cycle on a static bike, or stretching exercises—can help. This exercise can have the added benefit of raising body temperature, so you make the transition from warm to cooler when you enter your bed.

Sleeping Through Your Nose

Breathing probably ranks even higher than sleeping as something most of us take for granted. Yet getting our breathing right while we sleep is vital if we want to transition undisturbed through our sleep cycles. Common disorders such as snoring and sleep apnea—in which the sufferer stops breathing repeatedly during the night and their brain's oxygen warning light wakes them each time (the patient won't even remember this in the morning; it's often a partner who first notices it)—can disrupt our sleep significantly, as well as that of anyone sharing a bed with us, and both of these issues stem from our breathing.

In his excellent book *The Oxygen Advantage*, something of a bible on nose-breathing, Patrick McKeown writes, "Breathing through the mouth has been proven to significantly increase the number of occurrences of snoring and obstructive sleep apnea. . . . As any child is aware, the nose is made for breathing, the mouth for eating."

Breathing through our nose seems simple enough, and there is a host of health benefits that come with adopting this method, but it's how we breathe at night that matters to us. If you wake up with a dry mouth and almost always take a drink of water to bed with you, it suggests you breathe through your mouth when you sleep. A moist mouth on waking would suggest you breathe through your nose. So how can we try to influence something that happens automatically when we're asleep?

If you've ever seen cyclists or runners with what looks like a bandage on their nose, then you've seen the answer. As part of our pre-sleep routine, we can put a Breathe Right nasal strip on our nose; the strip dilates the nasal passages and encourages us to continue breathing through our nose. More advanced products, such as the Turbine or Mute Nasal Dilators by Rhinomed, go inside the nose and open up the airways that way and are used by a growing number of elite athletes. Use the one you prefer. It's advisable to put the product on and breathe through it for a period before you go to bed to get used to it, and you can practice with it anytime—while traveling to work, at your desk, in the gym—to make nose-breathing natural for you.

Patrick McKeown goes one step further: he wears a Breathe Right strip and tapes his mouth shut with a light, hypoallergenic medical tape to ensure that he breathes through his nose at night. Patrick's quality of sleep improved immeasurably when he adopted this method, and it is one he recommends to his clients—once they've been assured that they won't suffocate in their sleep, of course. (It's perfectly safe.) A product called SleepQ+, a lip-seal gel innovated by Rob Davies of RespiraCorp, which lightly seals the mouth to promote nose-breathing at night, promises to revolutionize this practice.

Post-Sleep

If your pre-sleep is everything you do to prepare yourself to get the best quality of sleep, then your post-sleep is your routine to make sure all of that work and the subsequent hours spent asleep have not been wasted. A good post-sleep routine will help you move from a sleep state to a fully awake state, so that you can manage your day positively, and it will even set you up in the best way possible for when you go to bed that night.

Again, ninety minutes can seem like a long time to set aside in the morning, but this can include your journey to work. Postsleep, of course, begins with the anchor of the R90 technique, the constant wake time—but the trappings of modern life immediately provide an obstacle to our biological needs.

The Return of the Tech

If a professional athlete wakes up, checks their phone immediately, sees a tweet they don't like the look of, and starts responding in anger when they're not awake enough to do so rationally, they could be opening a can of worms that will take up the rest of their day. They might even be waking up to an unwanted story in the papers the following morning.

I won't check notifications and alerts on my phone the instant I wake up because I know that I'm not in the right state to deal with anything properly. You wouldn't want to respond to a message when you were drunk, would you? We're not quite with it when we wake, and our levels of cortisol—a hormone we produce in response to stress—are at their highest shortly after waking. We don't need to make them any higher or keep them up throughout the day, throwing our rhythms out of sync. The first part of your waking day doesn't have to be a potentially stressful one.

So it's best to keep your phone out of your room overnight. Have a standard alarm clock or, better yet, a dawn simulator to wake you up, so that the first thing you do in the morning is in keeping with your circadian rhythms. Then you should open the curtains or blinds and get the daylight flooding into you. This raises your alertness, helps set your body clock, and allows you to make the final hormone shift from melatonin to serotonin. It puts you in a better position than you were in even just a few minutes before to deal with whatever is waiting for you on the phone.

Ideally, you would leave your phone and other devices alone until later in the morning, after you've fueled and hydrated, but at the very least you should make sure it is not the first thing you do when you wake. Just as with technology at night, we can train ourselves to have a break from it in the morning. You could set your alarm on your phone to go off fifteen minutes after you get up so that you don't touch it until then. You could then increase that to twenty minutes, and so on. Ninety minutes tech-free at the start of the day is a lot to ask of some people, but fifteen minutes is better than nothing—it's that much closer to being in a full wake state.

Breakfast of Champions

"Breakfast is the most important meal of the day" is a well-worn cliché, and it might have certain breakfast-skipping PM chronotypes rolling their eyes. Let me put it another way: there is not a single athlete I have ever worked with who does not eat breakfast, regardless of their chronotype. They simply wouldn't be able to do what they do without it.

Having some breakfast gives us the fuel we need to start our day. If you had your evening meal at 8 p.m. the night before and then woke up at 7 a.m., you haven't eaten anything for eleven hours. If you're the kind of person who isn't hungry right after you get up, try to have something to eat in those first ninety minutes after waking, even if it's just something small, such as a few bites of toast, some sips of a smoothie, or a nibble of fruit. Do it every day, and you will soon find yourself eating the whole slice of toast or piece of fruit and slurping the last of the smoothie.

Eating breakfast gives us fuel for the day and ensures that we then get hungry again at lunchtime, and later at dinnertime. In other words, we're getting hungry at the right times, instead of wanting to snack on food that isn't good for us here and there and feeling tired and sluggish.

Breakfast doesn't have to be a time-consuming ritual: toast, cereal, and fruit are all quick to make and consume. Take some fluid on and get hydrated too. If you have the time and the re-sources, eat your breakfast outside when the weather allows, or eat in a daylight-filled room, so that the sun can do its bit to wake you up too. If it's dark and the middle of winter, eat your break-fast by the light of a daylight lamp instead of the artificial light in the kitchen. It's all too easy in the morning to eat something hurriedly with the curtains closed before dashing off to work.

Some of us love nothing more than a cup of tea or coffee to start our day. When caffeine is used in moderation, this is a per-fectly acceptable part of a post-sleep routine. We use caffeine in sports because it's a fantastic performance enhancer, but we use it carefully. Having too much caffeine when you wake imme-diately puts pressure on that upper limit of 400 milligrams per day. Daylight, hydration, and fuel will all help your body wake up in good time if you let them, and they won't make you crash later in the day. Remember, sleep quality is all about what you do from the point of waking.

Exercise

Exercise is an excellent aspect to incorporate into a post-sleep routine. There are those who swear by an early-morning run, swim, or gym session before work, but it doesn't have to be that strenuous. A walk, a little gentle yoga, or some Pilates to ease your body into the day, or walking or riding a bicycle to work if you're lucky enough to be able to do so, are all good ways to spend part of your post-sleep routine. If the exercise is outdoors, then all the better. You'll benefit from the sunlight waking you up, boosting your serotonin levels, and setting your biological clock, which is the kind of post-sleep activity that will help you sleep at night as well as benefit your waking day. For the increas-ing number of home workers we're seeing in society as working habits change (3.7 million employees in the United States now work from home at least half the time, a 103 percent increase since 2005),[3] going for a walk outside, to get some fresh air and sunlight, is a good thing to incorporate into your routine before you start work.

Gentle Mental Challenge

Getting the brain in gear in the morning can be a gradual process, so some simple acts of mental stimulation, such as listening to the radio, ironing a shirt, or doing odd jobs around the house, can help. Reading a book, taking in the news, or listening to a podcast on the way to work are all good ways to begin engaging with the world.

Chronotype

Understandably, chronotypes have a big part to play in our mornings. Post-sleep routines are more important for PMers because the AMers, whose last cycles of sleep before waking will be lighter, are at their best in the mornings anyway. Although it may sound counterintuitive when it could mean more time in bed for them, the closer to ninety minutes that a PMer is able to dedicate to post-sleep, the better. Be aware of colleagues with opposite chronotypes who may run you ragged in the morning and you them later, or vice versa. Get a daylight lamp on your desk to compensate.

Spending the Day in Bed

If you like sleeping in on your days off, the constant wake time in the R90 program is likely to be the first thing you'll sacrifice when you're in the mood for a day in bed with Netflix after a particularly tough week at work (or a late night out). But there's no need—you can still incorporate these things into your life while maintaining some kind of harmony with your body clock.

You should still set your alarm and get up at your constant wake time, and then do those aspects of your post-sleep routine you can muster. You will probably skip the exercise, but you can still go to the bathroom on waking, soak up some daylight, and have your breakfast. Then you can go back to bed. This way you're doing what you can to be in tune with your circadian rhythms, while also doing what you want to do—you're not making great sacrifices or depriving yourself of enjoyment to stick to the R90 program. Even professional sports people have days like these (usually *after* an event, of course), and sometimes there's nothing better for us than a movie marathon from under the covers—as long as we're managing it and not allowing it to disrupt our natural routine too much. It is important to try to associate only recovery activities with our bedroom as much as possible.

Sleep Efficiently

We can't control what we do while we're asleep, but we can control everything we do leading up to it and afterward. Incorporating pre- and post-sleep routines into our lives can appear difficult at first, particularly when our time already feels pinched, but through some subtle changes to our schedules we can all find ways to do it.

The benefits can be summed up in one word: efficiency. Our pre-sleep routine gets us prepared to enter our sleep cycles, so we can get the very best quality of recovery during our time in bed—even if that time is truncated because of our lifestyle. It gives us the flexibility and freedom to go to bed later when needed, confident that we can download our day and do our best to dispel any lingering unhelpful thoughts so that we won't waste our valuable time on not sleeping.

Our post-sleep routine enables us to be more efficient in our waking day. By taking the time to apply it, we are able to arrive at work or social engagements more prepared and alert, so that we're getting the maximum out of these activities and putting the most we can back into them. We can arrive at our 9 a.m. appointments feeling sharp instead of rushed and overstimulated on caffeine.

By adopting a post-sleep routine, we can start to feel empowered to make decisions that will preserve that time. If your constant wake time is 7:30 a.m. and someone suggests an 8:30 a.m. meeting, you can politely suggest 9 a.m. instead, so you can have your ninety minutes to get yourself ready. If they can't budge, then sixty minutes is acceptable as a post-sleep routine, but anything less—such as for an 8 a.m. meeting—is too short and counterproductive, in which case you'd move a whole cycle back and get up at 6. These decisions can then start to feed into other aspects of your life.

If you have a plane to catch and need to drive to the airport early in the morning, you have a decision to make. Either you can jump out of bed, get dressed, and drive there, or you can make a one-time choice to bring your wake time back one cycle (from 7:30 to 6 a.m.). If you choose the latter, you're more likely to stick to the speed limit because you're not feeling rushed and you are more alert, despite getting up earlier. You're fueled and hydrated, you've used the bathroom, you've exercised, and you've exposed yourself to daylight (whether that's naturally or through a daylight lamp)—all the things your body wants to do instead of leaping straight into a car and driving. Once you get to the airport, you can hold a conversation more competently. If you don't like the look of something when you're at the airport—an unattended bag, for example—you can make a better decision as to what to do about it.

In sports, these decisions can produce microscopic advantages in real time—a couple of thousandths of a second in a race—which might make all the difference. For a PMer sprinter competing earlier in the day, when they're not quite at their best, a good post-sleep routine could be the difference between snatching the bronze medal at the finish line and coming in fourth, outside of the medals. It might mean an athlete having the alertness to know not to push it any more in training, while their rival without an effective post-sleep routine pulls up with a calf strain, and their race is over before they've even reached the starting line.

PRE- AND POST-SLEEP ROUTINES:
SEVEN STEPS TO SLEEP SMARTER

1. Pre- and post-sleep routines directly affect the quality of your sleep and waking day. Value them as the important activities they are, and you'll be more efficient all day and night.

2. Take breaks from technology during the day as a reward and training for body and mind.

3. Post-sleep is vitally important for PMers if they want to keep up with the AMers. Don't skip this in favor of hitting the snooze button.

4. Don't text drunk! Raise your alertness before you reach for your phone.

5. Moving your body from warm to cooler helps trigger the natural drop in body temperature associated with sleep. A quick warm rinse under the shower and a cooler sleeping environment will achieve this.

6. Declutter your environment and mind and download your day before bed, so you don't lie awake thinking when you could be asleep.

7. Pre-sleep is about shutting down—nose-breathing, relaxing, light to dark—while post-sleep is about starting up in an unrushed way. These periods belong to you and no one else.

FIVE

Time Out!

Redefining Naps: Activity and Recovery Harmony

Welcome to your Friday afternoon post-lunch meeting. The sun slants into the warm room through the half-closed blinds, illuminating the dust hovering in the air. Your pizza lunch still sits heavily in your stomach, and you try to listen to the presenter's voice describing the slides while the projector whirrs soothingly in the background. Your eyelids are becoming heavy just as . . .

Whoa! You snap awake. How long were you out for? You look around the table for disapproving stares, a colleague's stifled grin, but instead all eyes are on the presenter. What a relief. It must have been only a matter of seconds. You got away with it this time, but it's a signal that you need to really concentrate on the meeting now. You turn toward the presenter, pick your pen up from the table, and do your best to focus on what's being said, really giving it your all.

And then it happens again.

The Afternoon Slump

To some it's the corporate graveyard slot, to others the post-lunch slump. Whatever you want to call it, this midday period when daytime fatigue kicks in, which the Spanish have traditionally indulged with their siestas while most of the rest of the world pushes on through with unproductive meetings and heavy doses of caffeine, is an all too familiar phenomenon in homes and workplaces across the planet. It is also the key to re-defining sleep as you know it.

In the R90 program thus far we have addressed your approach to sleeping at night, but if you really want to learn to do it like the elite athletes I work with, you must learn to unlock the hours in the day as well. It is here that we will learn to think not in terms of sleep but, instead, of the process of mental and physical *recovery*.

Recovery is a twenty-four-hours-a-day, seven-days-a-week commitment, and by using the daylight hours in addition to your nocturnal approach you will be able to give your mind and body the opportunity to continually reboot while dealing with the demands of modern life.

The second natural recovery period at midday is where we start, as this is the biggest and most effective natural window to claim back a cycle we have missed out on at night, to prepare us for a potential later evening ahead, and to use in harmony with our nocturnal cycles as part of our weekly sleep-wake routine. By using this time to have an afternoon nap, we can begin to maximize all the hours in the day in order to perform better.

Don't be put off if you're not a napper. The kind of napping you're probably familiar with is part of the old-school approach to sleep. We don't call them naps in sports—we call them controlled recovery periods (CRPs). We don't nod off indiscriminately. We take ownership of these opportunities during the day and extract the maximum benefits from them. Just like the CEOs of leading corporations and some of the most successful figures in the arts and entertainment do. Just like you can, even if you think you can't sleep during the day, because *anyone* can learn to use a controlled recovery period, and it's something *everyone* should learn to do.

When Urge and Need Collide

History is littered with famous afternoon nappers, such as Winston Churchill, Napoleon Bonaparte, and Bill Clinton, and the siesta period is still observed in countries all over the world, not only in Spain but elsewhere in the Mediterranean and in the tropics and subtropics. If we look at the hunter-gatherer communities that still exist today—the closest we can get to looking directly at how we might have lived thousands of years ago, and certainly easier than relocating to an uninhabited island to find out ourselves—we can see that polyphasic sleep is very much the norm. Carol Worthman, professor of anthropology at Emory University, studied non-Westernized people in places like Botswana, Zaire, Paraguay, and Indonesia, and reported: "Sleep is a very fluid state. They sleep when they feel like it—during the day, in the evening, in the dead of night."[1]

The patterns of the internal sleep regulators in our bodies show that sleeping in a polyphasic way is perfectly natural. In Chapter 1, we talked about how our sleep is regulated by our circadian rhythms (our *urge* to sleep) and our building sleep pressure (our *need* to sleep). The main sleep window occurs at night, when our circadian urge climbs (it peaks at around 2–3 a.m.) and intersects with our high need for sleep.

But in the midafternoon—between 1 and 3 p.m. for most people, or a little later for some PM chronotypes—something interesting happens. Our sleep pressure builds steadily, as expected, but our circadian rhythm spikes upward from its morning low, producing an increased urge to sleep that coincides with quite a high need as the day goes on. The result is another sleep window.

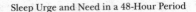

Sleep Urge and Need in a 48-Hour Period

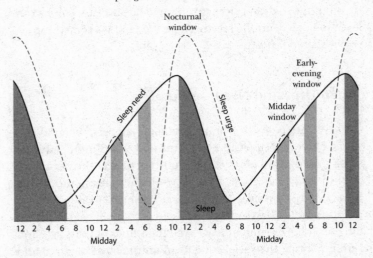

This window is a perfect opportunity to fit in either a full ninety-minute cycle or a thirty-minute controlled recovery period perfectly in harmony with our body's urge and need. When I'm addressing an athlete's schedule, this midday period is used to compensate for fewer cycles at night, whether that's the night before or in anticipation of the night ahead. When tallying up the cycles for the week, getting one in here—either thirty or ninety minutes—counts toward the total for the week.

The Power of the Nap

The power of the nap cannot be ignored. A study conducted at the University of Düsseldorf has shown that even very short naps enhance memory processing,[2] while a NASA study looking at pilots on long flights reported, "Naps can maintain or improve subsequent performance, physiological and subjective alertness, and mood."[3] One of the authors of that report, Mark

Rosekind, head of the National Highway Traffic Safety Administration, has said that "a twenty-six-minute nap improves performance in pilots by 34 percent and alertness by 54 percent."[4]

Naps are of critical importance to pilots flying long haul—they fit one in while the co-pilot takes over, later reaping the benefits of improved alertness. We'd all like a pilot to be at their best when it's time to land. They are a significant personal performance enhancer for athletes too, and they can have the same benefits for anyone. Given the demands on our lives, sleeping at night is often the first thing to suffer, and we have to find ways of managing this. But we also have to find ways of fitting CRPs into our own schedules, as sleeping during the day still isn't regarded favorably by many employers.

An elite athlete is more likely to enjoy the luxury of capitalizing on a full ninety-minute cycle in this period, as physical recovery is a very real and accepted part of their job. They (usually) don't have a supervisor wondering where on earth they've disappeared to for ninety minutes.

A ninety-minute cycle has a potential drawback immediately afterward, in the form of sleep inertia, which is the groggy, disoriented feeling on waking. This is important to bear in mind when scheduling these controlled recovery periods. If an Olympic athlete is competing in the evening, then they will have the time to overcome any potential sleep inertia and enjoy the benefits of this period of sleep; if they're competing earlier, then we would look at either a thirty-minute nap period or none at all.

The thirty-minute option is likely to be the most practical for the rest of us. While studies have shown that thirty-minute naps can produce sleep inertia, as it is possible to reach deep sleep over this period of time, this is of very little consequence in my experience and won't be a factor at all if you do it like the athletes I work with.[5] Take a dose of caffeine beforehand—espresso is a good quick fix—so that it takes effect toward the end of your CRP. Caffeine takes about twenty minutes to affect the body, and it is a useful performance enhancer in controlled doses. Try not to consume your caffeine as a leisurely latte, as you might find the caffeine is already taking effect as you begin your CRP, and be aware of the amount of caffeine you have already consumed. If you are hovering around the 400-milligram daily maximum, go without the little dose of caffeine. A daylight lamp on your desk or getting out into natural daylight will also see you through any inertia very quickly, so that you will enjoy all the benefits of a controlled recovery period, just like those who took the twenty-six-minute naps in the NASA study.

How to Take a Controlled Recovery Period

Branding the midafternoon snooze as the "power nap" has allowed the practice to shed some of its bad reputation in the corporate world. The effectiveness of these short restorative sleeps has been acknowledged by many companies, which provide facilities for their staff to take a power nap in the afternoon. These facilities can range from the relatively basic to the space-age, with piped-in whale songs and aromatherapy. The truth is, you don't need any of this.

When I was working with Manchester United in the late 1990s, the club introduced double training sessions in the preseason for the first time. I suggested providing facilities for the players in which they could relax and have a CRP between sessions to improve their recovery from the first training session and prepare them better for the second. Both Alex Ferguson and the head physical therapist, Rob Swire, supported the idea, so we introduced what was probably the world's first ever training-facility recovery room. We found a suitable room that could accommodate up to twelve players at a time, put in some single-sleeper couches, and coached the players on how to use the space. It was all very basic—no whale songs or aromatherapy—but it did the job. It was a key step toward where we are today with sleep recovery, and the players of one of the most successful teams in the club's history—and in the entire history of professional soccer, for that matter—took full advantage of it by keeping their minds open to something as radical as daytime sleeping.

The truth is that we can nap anywhere. Most of us will have experienced nodding off in a meeting or on a packed subway, and if we can do it there, then we can certainly try it in a more controlled environment. Even if you don't work for the kind of employer that has made naps part of its employee well-being program, you can find a space somewhere to do it: an unused office or meeting room, a quiet corner in the communal kitchen, the sofa in the staff room, or even on a park bench when the weather permits. It's not like going to sleep at night, so if you're unable to find somewhere to lie down comfortably, do it sitting up. I've even known of people locking themselves away in a bathroom stall for an afternoon nap, and pilots do it in their cockpit seat while flying at over 500 mph at 35,000 feet.

You don't need to worry about people being around you either. Once you get good at this, they won't even be aware of what you're doing. But before we get ahead of ourselves, let's just start by finding a spot where you can get yourself comfortable at some point during this afternoon period. If you work from home, don't use your bed for this; use a sofa or armchair, and keep your bed for sleeping in at night or for a full ninety-minute afternoon cycle. Set your phone to "do not disturb" if possible, just so you won't be interrupted by the sound of an incoming notification or message, and set the alarm for, ideally, thirty minutes. If you have less time, set it for whatever you have—shorter naps are beneficial too.

Then close your eyes and just let go. Easier said than done, you might be thinking. Some people will be able to do this and fall asleep promptly. They might wake up ten or twenty minutes later, or it might be their alarm that wakes them. Others, those who steadfastly claim that they simply "can't nap," won't be able to fall asleep. But this is one of the revelatory things about this process for those people: *it doesn't matter.*

Really, it does not matter if you don't actually enter a sleep state. What is important is that you use this period to close your eyes and disconnect from your world for a while. Falling asleep is great, but so is catching that place on the verge of sleep, when you're not quite awake but not quite asleep either, and so too is that point of daydreaming when you're not really thinking about anything at all, when your mind is just a great big blank.

There are tools that can help with this: meditation practices, mindfulness apps, and all sorts of other things that you can use to just take yourself away from it all. By doing this, we're able to step away from the stresses and strains of our day, which enables us to get a head start on some of the downloading that we will do later as part of our pre-sleep routine. With the focus of our conscious mind diffused and its energies spread elsewhere, we're able to absorb and file away the events of our day so far.

The brain is a powerful tool that can be trained to do all kinds of remarkable things. Through regularly putting ourselves in a position to take advantage of this midafternoon slump, even those who maintain that they "can't nap" will find themselves becoming better at it. When used in conjunction with a shorter-cycle routine at night, when this period of fatigue will be even more pronounced, they might find themselves drifting off to sleep, even if it's just for a few minutes, which is enough for our brains to begin processing memories. After a nap, take five minutes to become aware of your surroundings, hydrate, and get some daylight on you if possible. Your heightened mood and alertness, as well as the dip in your need for sleep, will benefit you throughout the rest of the afternoon—and even into the evening.

The Early-Evening Recovery Period

For those unable to capitalize on the midday recovery period, another opportunity presents itself later in the day. If you've ever traveled home from work and caught yourself nodding off, or you've arrived home in the early evening and drifted off in front of the television for a short while, you'll already be familiar with this slot.

Sleeping twice in the night is not without precedent. Historian Roger Ekirch presented evidence in his book *At Day's Close: A History of Nighttime* that we once slept in two distinct chunks, the first after dusk and the second through to dawn after a couple of hours spent awake in the middle of the night. However, this was before artificial lighting opened up the potential of our evenings and the industrial revolution made segmented sleep seem like a waste of time in a productivity-driven society.

I am not for a second suggesting we return to this. The night is very much alive for us today, and none of us want to miss a good evening out if we can help it. What I am suggesting is capitalizing on a time in the early evening, somewhere between 5 and 7 p.m. (or a little later for some PM chronotypes), when our *need* for sleep is high, particularly if we've had less than normal the night previously, even if our urge is dipping. This window can be used for a thirty-minute controlled recovery period if the midday window has been missed; however, a ninety-minute cycle is likely to interfere with your nocturnal sleep later.

This window is more practical for many people, particularly those working 9–5 jobs. While they might struggle to fit in a midday CRP due to work commitments, or they simply don't work in an environment conducive to being able to take a suitable break, this early-evening window can be convenient: they can come home from work (often exhausted), have their CRP, and then get more out of their evening.

The early-evening period is steeped in the cliché of an old man with his pipe and slippers nodding off with the newspaper in his lap. Times have changed, though, and this recovery window is an opportunity to redefine this tired old image. There is a myth surrounding sleep that says our need for it declines as we get older. In fact, while our ability to sleep efficiently declines with age, the amount we need does not.

The more mature CEO of a business who wants to keep going for as long as possible should take note of this. We naturally become more polyphasic in our sleep as we get older, so instead of scheduling meetings and overstimulating to push through these periods, use them to recharge yourself. If you're feeling sleepy in this time slot, take control of it. Find a quiet place, set the alarm on your device for thirty minutes, and close your eyes. The improvements to your performance will far outweigh those any cup of coffee would have, and you'll be adding to your diminishing and increasingly fragmented cycles at night. If you tend to nod off in this period on the sofa at home, take control of this too: take yourself off to a quiet place, set the alarm, and have your controlled recovery period so that you get the maximum benefit out of it.

If you miss out on the midday period and instead anticipate using this evening slot to take a CRP, you still have to get through the afternoon. This is where some manipulation of your daytime schedule is in order, if your job permits it, so that you're not exposing yourself to anything too taxing when you know you're in a slump. You could try to avoid meetings in the post-lunch period, or at least control the times of any you schedule yourself. If you can manipulate things so that your least demanding tasks are around this period—some filing or photocopying, or putting together the elements of a report you've already done the hard work on—then all the better. And if there is any aspect of your job that involves being outside, such as going to the bank or the post office, try to make it around here.

Daylight, as always, is our friend when it comes to giving us a boost, and it is the reason you should not spend your entire lunch break eating at your desk. If you do eat at your desk, try to get outside for some daylight and fresh air instead of just working straight through. If you can't manage this, you (or your company) could invest in a daylight lamp to give you a boost at your desk, or you could use a product such as Valkee's Human Charger, which, to the casual observer, will look like you're listening to your tunes on your headphones as you work. In fact, it delivers light therapy to your pineal gland through your ears.

Wherever you work, get some light on you in this period. Your productivity is down and you need a break and a boost here to help you through the midafternoon slump.

Take a Break

Opening up these two windows of time during the day will give you the confidence to take some of the pressure off your sleep. It will allow you to go to bed later and not worry as much about whether you're getting enough sleep; if you're awake in the night, there's reassurance to be found in knowing that you can schedule a CRP the next day. These periods can't replace your nocturnal sleep in the long term, which is why the R90 program advises that you get your ideal routine in at least four times in a week, but they can work in harmony with your body's rhythms to augment your cycles at night, strengthen your recovery, and help your mood and productivity remain high.

Sleep is not just about physical sleep; it is about giving the mind the opportunity to recover throughout a twenty-four-hour process. Naps open up these two windows in the day, but we must also look to tap into even smaller windows more regularly throughout our day if we are to give our minds and our bodies the opportunity to perform at their best.

Using breaks is a vital part of the approach. In sports, the physical necessity is obvious: if we're putting an athlete through a particularly lung-busting training routine, they'll need to recover before they attempt the next part of their session. But there is a mental need that's every bit as important. We require regular breaks to help consolidate information and because our concentration won't hold without them. Elite performers are just like the rest of us in this: they get distracted—bored, even. The concentration of any elite athlete will eventually waver if they continue doing a task for too long.

Swedish psychologist K. Anders Ericsson, whose research formed the basis of the famous notion that ten thousand hours of deliberate practice is required for world-class mastery of a skill, wrote: "Expert performers from many domains engage in practice without rest for only around an hour. . . . Elite musicians and athletes report that the factor that limits their deliberate practice is primarily an inability to sustain the level of concentration that is necessary."[6]

While most of us might not look at what we do in our day-to-day lives as something so grand as "deliberate practice," the lesson still holds. We can't sustain the levels of concentration we need when we're working, so eventually, without a break, we're going to become less efficient. We're going to become fatigued and frustrated.

Take a break. If you're able to step away from your work every hour, then you should do so, but for many people this isn't tenable. However, if we look at recovery in ninety-minute segments, as we do with the R90 approach, it becomes a bit more possible. Most of us who work in an office can find a reason to get away from our desks every ninety minutes, and even if you work in a shop, on a factory floor, or somewhere more restrictive of your time, taking a break every ninety minutes is going to be easier than doing it every hour.

No time for a break? Then *make* time. You're going to be more efficient for having one, with refreshed levels of concentration for the tasks at hand. It doesn't have to be a major break. Go and make a cup of coffee or tea (consider something decaf!); go to the bathroom (even if you don't really need it); head outside for a couple of minutes; get up and talk to a colleague or make a phone call. It doesn't really matter—the point is that you're moving away from the environment and mental state you work in to give your mind a little recovery window. If you sit at a desk all day, it will do your body some good to get away from it too.

Start making little adjustments that will make it easier for you. No one is going to stop you from getting a drink of water, so instead of filling up a two-liter bottle and keeping it on your desk, just have a glass of water that needs to be refilled more regularly.

During these breaks, we can tap into what we try to do when we nap, which is to disassociate our thoughts from our environment and just tune out for a little while. These "mind breaks" every ninety minutes will improve your performance immediately after taking them, reduce stress levels, and will accumulate during the course of the day to prevent you from feeling quite so tired in the afternoon and early evening.[7] They are also contributing to the downloading of your day, allowing you to subconsciously absorb and file away what you've been doing. A break every ninety minutes, along with a controlled recovery period when necessary—they all add up.

With a bit of practice, you'll be able to take advantage of moments in meetings or group conversations in which you're not heavily involved to just step back and take a little mind break. You're effectively napping with your eyes open in a room full of people; they have no idea what you are doing. You could go talk to a colleague about last night's baseball game or what they watched on television, something that isn't fully demanding of your attention, and do it there. Something comfortable and effort-free to talk about is a nice break for the mind—and you can always drift away in your own head if the person you're talking to is going on and on.

You can use your headphones at your desk to listen to a meditation app or something else that will help you switch off for a minute or two. I carry around with me a polished stone with some very strong associations for me; when I need to switch off in this way, I can reach into my pocket, hold it in my hand, and just drift away for a while, giving my mind the opportunity to recover. You might even be talking to me while I'm doing it—you just won't have a clue.

Set the timer on your phone for every ninety minutes so you don't forget to take a break. This will start to give you a sense of what ninety minutes feels like, and before long you won't need the timer anymore—you'll naturally feel that it's time to briefly get away from what you're doing.

You'll soon see that your whole day—not just your night—can be broken up into cycles of ninety minutes. You can use these to get some harmony between your periods of activity and recovery. With your cycles at night, your pre- and post-sleep routines, your controlled recovery periods, and these breaks, your day no longer looks like one long stretch of go, go, go before you crash into bed for *maybe* eight hours, probably less, and do it all again.

You can start to get creative with these breaks, using them to benefit other elements of the Key Sleep Recovery Indicators. You could take a break from your technology every ninety minutes. Like the breaks from it you take to benefit your pre- and post-sleep routines, make them a reward for your body and mind. Start with just five minutes, but try to work up to twenty, so that in every ninety minutes you are only spending seventy connected to email, social media, alerts, and messages. If during one of these periods you get the urge to send a message, write it down instead and send it later. You aren't going to lose friends or status at work because you take twenty minutes to reply to emails at certain times of the day, and the confidence you gain from your ability to take these breaks is all good training for when it's time to pare back your tech use during your pre-sleep routine later.

If You Don't Snooze, You'll Lose

Naps have gotten bad press, with their practitioners often labeled as lazy or work-shy, and even the Spanish are looking at phasing out their siesta. Many companies have made strides in their well-being programs, but too many are still stuck in the dark ages when it comes to attitudes toward mental and physical recovery, and this has to stop. The awful phrase "you snooze, you lose" is beloved of a certain type of opportunity-grabbing businessperson, but you'll be stuck along with these dinosaurs in the group labeled "burnout" if you don't adopt updated ideas about sleep and recovery. When it comes to recovery, if you *don't* snooze, you will lose eventually.

The National Highway Traffic Safety Administration estimates that there are an average of 83,000 crashes related to drowsy driving each year in the United States; the Massachusetts Special Commission on Drowsy Driving estimates there could be as many as 1.2 million.[8] Another report has highlighted the correlation between time of day and traffic accidents where sleep has been a factor.[9] No surprise to learn that they're most likely to occur between 2 and 6 a.m. and in the midafternoon slump between 2 and 4 p.m.—even when no sleep deprivation has occurred.

Tiredness kills—and it kills performance too. We use controlled recovery periods in elite sports, where the athletes are anything but "lazy" or "work-shy," and, as K. Anders Ericsson points out, elite performers in other fields, such as famous writers and musicians, have an "increased tendency to take recuperative naps."[10]

In other words, if you want to learn from the elite, it's time to learn to take a break and recover. It is time for corporations to redefine their culture by minimizing meetings during the post-lunch slump, offering employees legitimate opportunities to get away from their work, promoting regular breaks, and providing the facilities and encouragement for staff to take a controlled recovery period. Take a leaf from the book of tech giants like Google, whose flexible working hours and culture allow it to assert a bold workplace philosophy: "To create the happiest, most productive workforce in the world."

Start taking these breaks seriously, because companies will enjoy the benefits of increased productivity and happiness in the long term—and so will you.

ACTIVITY AND RECOVERY HARMONY: SEVEN STEPS TO SLEEP SMARTER

1. A controlled recovery period during the midday window (1–3 p.m.) is the perfect way to supplement your nocturnal cycles in harmony with your circadian rhythms.

2. The early evening (5–7 p.m.) is the next-best opportunity, as the need is high—but limit this one to thirty minutes maximum so it won't affect your sleep at night.

3. Can't sleep in the day? It doesn't matter—just spend thirty minutes switching off and disconnecting from the world.

4. Take breaks at least every ninety minutes to refresh your mind and your concentration levels. Avoid technology during these windows, so that you're not spending a whole ninety minutes connected.

5. Get rid of any preconceived notions of daytime sleepers being "lazy," and work to provide a culture where CRPs and breaks are accepted. If you don't snooze, you'll lose.

6. Use meditation apps, try mindfulness techniques, or hold an item of personal value to help you slip away from your immediate environment.

7. If you really can't get away, manipulate your day so that you're not caught doing anything too taxing in the mid-afternoon slump.

SIX

The Sleep Kit

Reinventing the Bed

A young and ambitious couple has just bought a condo to-gether. After years spent sleeping on whatever came with their furnished rented accommodation, they are buying a queen-size bed frame and mattress for the first time.

They have done some research, looking up the "top tips" on various websites. They know that they need to spend as much money as they can on the mattress because these top tips have told them so; it's an investment because a good one should last ten years. Get memory foam, choose pocketed coils, spend more on the mattress than the frame—they feel they know the basics, and they know their budget.

They undo it all immediately by buying a stylish bed frame online, blowing half their budget in the process. But even though they can buy a mattress online, that's not what the top tips suggest. They know they need to try it out. So they enter the mattress store with the express intention of lying on some mattresses for a whole five or ten minutes to get a feel for them.

The salesperson greets them, immediately checking out the expensive watch, the tailored jacket, the designer handbag, and thinks, *Let's start these guys out on a $2,000 mattress.* He shows them a pocketed-coil orthopedic mattress, top of the line. "It will do wonders for your posture," says the salesperson, smiling. It's got all sorts of bells and whistles and thousands of coils, but he can see a look of discomfort on their faces when he tells them the price, so he takes them down to the $1,500 option, and then the $1,000 option.

They bounce around on the beds, then lie on their backs on them for a couple of minutes, assuming what they imagine to be their sleeping position, using the pillows provided. "Go ahead, get right in and give it a try," says the salesperson. They get in, laughing, and close their eyes in the middle of the brightly lit store.

The fun eventually comes to an end, however, and now it's time to make a decision.

"Which one felt the most comfortable to you?"

"I'm not sure. Maybe the second one? It was nice and firm, but not *too* firm."

The second option is $500 over their budget, but it's the middle-priced choice and they feel reassured by the fact that it has more coils than the cheapest. *That's got to count for something*, they think. They turn to the salesperson and say together, "We'll take this one."

"Excellent choice," says the salesperson, beaming.

The couple walks out of the shop having spent $500 more than they intended to. They have their queen mattress, and they're grateful that they won't have to do *that* again for another ten years.

But did they make the right decision?

The Mattress-Buying Blind Side

Can you think of another purchase involving such a significant amount of money that you would walk into so blind? Would you buy a car armed with nothing but some "top tips" from a newspaper puff piece—or from the retailer itself? You're about to spend a third of your life on this thing.

Yet millions of people do exactly the same every year. They walk blindly into a store, throw themselves on the mercy of the salespeople, and more often than not leave with something that will do the job but is unlikely to change their lives. They won't even know if they've got the right or wrong one because they don't know what the right or wrong one is.

We buy beds and mattresses infrequently—a good one should last us ten years, we're told—so few of us are armed with much up-to-date, reliable information. Why would we be? Beds are about style, and a mattress is just something most of us take for granted. When it comes to buying a new one, we will do a bit of cursory research online—and there is a lot of contradictory advice on the Web, the bulk of which tells us that we need a "good mattress" without ever getting to the crux of what that actually means, and gives people all kinds of ideas about how much they should be spending and how long the mattress should last.

The bed retailers and manufacturers, meanwhile, are well aware of this. And I should know—I have worked in the industry, and indeed continue to work in it today, as I produce mattresses and bedding as well as sleep kits for athletes (more on those kits later).

The first thing to realize about the bedding industry is that there is little in the way of regulation beyond flammability standards. I could manufacture a mattress with the tensile strength of the coils ratcheted so high an elephant could sleep on it, put some high-density foam pads on top to make it firmer still, cover it in an attractive, faux-medical fabric with a label saying "orthopedic" on it, and go sell this in a store without anyone stopping me. Am I a doctor? Do I have any kind of orthopedic training? Have I put the mattress through a series of tests to determine its orthopedic properties? All I've done is make the hardest mattress I possibly can, and there is nothing to prevent me from making the claim that it has beneficial qualities.

I might then make sure it has 2,000 coils in it, because my competitor has a 1,500-spring mattress and 2,000 sounds better than 1,500. It becomes like an arms race, with manufacturers making smaller coils so they can fit more in. You're not comparing apples with apples here, but few of us ask these questions. And what if you only really need fifty coils anyway? Unless we have something to gauge a number against, what use is it? The young couple didn't stop to interrogate the data they were being provided with; they simply assumed more is better. They also didn't take notice of the small print. The figure of 2,000 is likely to be the number in the king-size mattress, with fewer coils as you go down in size. Retailers won't always make this clear.

I would never send an athlete into one of these stores to buy a mattress. It would be like sending the best linebacker in the NFL into a discount sportswear store to buy his cleats. Athletes need to be armed with the right knowledge, or else I go with them—or I could simply make the product for them.

Gary Pallister was the soccer player with the back problem I helped at Manchester United when I first got involved with the club. He was a seasoned defender, but the years of playing professional soccer had taken their toll, and he suffered from a lot of lower-back strains and pain. Even in today's game, surgery for a spinal injury would be the very last resort, so instead they were wrapping him in cotton wool. Dave Fevre, the head physical therapist at the club, was treating Gary for a good length of time every day, and his training was reduced to a bare minimum. They were even considering stripping out seats on the team bus to install a lumbar-supporting chair-bed for him.

When I came in, we looked at what he was doing away from the club in terms of "dehabilitating rather than rehabilitating" the condition, to use Dave's words. Among other things, Gary's mattress was not good for his posture and was aggravating his condition. Shortly after we changed it, Dave started to see that Gary needed less treatment. He wasn't cured, not by any stretch of the imagination, but he was no longer aggravating his back, and the club didn't have to completely remodel the bus.

If an elite athlete goes into a shop and the salesperson recognizes them, they'll be taken straight to the very top end, for the most expensive mattresses of all. Thousands and thousands of dollars can be spent on a mattress, but it won't be spent in the quest to find the right one. It will be because the salesperson wants to sell them the most expensive one, with all of the latest marketing jargon.

One Size Fits All? (Again)

Earlier in the book, we discussed the eight-hours-of-sleep-per-night approach and the fallacy of applying a one-size-fits-all mentality to sleep. The same logic that applies to the amount of time you spend sleeping extends to the surface you spend that time on.

Take LeBron James, for example. He's six foot eight, very well built, and weighs about 250 pounds. There is no logic in thinking that the best mattress for him would be the same as that for four-time Olympic gold medalist gymnast Simone Biles, who stands around four foot eight and weighs in at around 105 pounds.

There is no acknowledgment of body profiles in the mattress industry. No salesperson will look you up and down and point you to your "size." Some brands will offer a variety of mattresses of differing firmness, but you could walk out of the store with any one of them, whether or not they're the right one. Some of the new fashionable brands, with clever marketing strategies behind them, only make one mattress. One mattress for *everyone*, any shape or weight. How does that work?

This doesn't happen when you buy footwear or an item of clothing. You buy the size that fits. So why should a mattress be any different? Like the small, medium, and large sizes in clothing, there are three main body types, with the extra-smalls and extra-larges at the extremes.

Ectomorph is a lean build, with narrow hips and pelvis and long arms and legs. They typically have less fat and muscle mass than the other profiles. Usain Bolt and Michael Phelps are good examples of this body profile. For a female example, take your pick from models Kate Moss and Cara Delevingne, or actress Diane Keaton.

Mesomorph is a medium body shape and build, with thick bones and muscles, a well-defined chest, and shoulders broader than the hips. Many professional athletes fit this body profile, with tennis players Rafael Nadal, Andre Agassi, or Björn Borg good male examples, and Venus Williams for a female.

Endomorph is a larger build, with wide shoulders and broader hips. Think actress Sofía Vergara, comedian Amy Schumer, or the singer Adele for the women, and the Hollywood actors Russell Crowe and Seth Rogen, and boxers Anthony Joshua and Muhammad Ali for the boys.

Naturally, there is crossover—it's a sliding scale, with some people a blend of meso and ecto and others on the endo-meso border. You can be tall or short, carrying a little extra weight or underweight, and still fit your profile. The characteristics of men and women differ too.

It makes clear sense that two people of the same height but of different body profiles are going to have different requirements in a sleeping surface. Their mattresses are going to need to give to different degrees to provide the requisite level of comfort. Partners complicate matters too, and where there is a difference in body profile, you go with the dominant one (so a meso and endo couple would go with the endo, an ecto and meso couple with the meso).

But before you rush off to check your body profile, there's a far easier, foolproof method to guarantee you're buying the right mattress. And it all starts with making sure you are sleeping in the correct position.

How to Sleep

So far we've looked at the preparation before and after sleep, organizing your time in bed according to your sleep cycles, and how to compensate for late nights. We've looked at what to do around your sleep—but we've been taking it for granted that, once you get into bed at night, you know *how* to sleep.

Just like the body profiles, there are three basic sleeping positions, and we're all familiar with them: *stomach, back,* and *side*. Again, these aren't three mutually exclusive positions—you can maneuver your limbs into all sorts of contortionist arrangements while you sleep to blur the lines, and a mountaineer at high altitude might wonder where "hanging in a bag from a sheer cliff" falls on the list. But for those of us getting into a bed at night, these are the three main positions.

Sleeping on our back is a popular option, with the postural benefit of keeping the back and neck aligned (provided you aren't sleeping on a pillow that interferes with this), but it makes us relax our throat and causes a narrowing of the airways. The British Snoring and Sleep Apnea Association says, "Individuals who sleep in the supine position (on the back) are more likely to snore or have increased apneas than those who sleep in the lateral position (on the side)." These are factors that are going to interfere with our sleep: they can take us out of a sleep cycle altogether or doom us to a night of light sleep. And they can do the same to our partners if we have them, not to mention cause resentment and put strains on a relationship. Lying on our back also leaves us feeling exposed and keeps our brain in a state of alert.

Sleeping on our stomach might help with snoring, but it comes with plenty of its own problems. Stomach-sleepers twist their spine into an unnatural position and, unless they're sleeping facedown into their pillow, which can become an aggravating factor in itself, their neck is being twisted too. Lower-back pain, neck ache, and all sorts of postural problems can stem from sleeping on your stomach. Furthermore, the postural problems caused by sitting in front of a computer all day and looking down at our smartphones and handheld devices can be exacerbated by stomach sleeping, with all of it adding up to neck and spine aggravation.

Sleeping on your side is the only sleeping position I recommend—but it might not be the side you currently sleep on. When the athletes I coach go to bed at night, they get into the fetal position on their *non-dominant* side, because this is the less used and therefore less sensitive side. In other words, if you're right-handed, you sleep on your left side, and vice versa. If you're genuinely ambidextrous, think about which side you would instinctively use to protect yourself.

The fetal position should involve a gentle bend at the knees and your arms out in front of you, gently folded. You should have a smooth, straight postural line through the neck, spine, and bottom. You want to remain in this position for as long as possible during the night. (You will, of course, move during the hours of sleep, but your mattress should allow you to adopt this position for longer periods.)

Your spine and neck are in a natural position, which won't cause any postural problems. Your chances of snoring or sleep apnea are reduced. Your brain likes this position because it feels that your body is secure—your dominant arm and leg are protecting your heart and other organs, and your genitals.

When I spent some time traveling around Europe, I would occasionally sleep overnight in a train station, having missed the last train that evening and with nowhere else to go. I would lie down on the ground—a particularly firm mattress—with my backpack for a pillow and my valuables tucked away in my inside jacket pocket, covered by my dominant arm. If anyone had tried to pickpocket me, I would have been able to defend myself with my strongest side. This kind of security, which allows us to fall asleep in an exposed and potentially problematic environment, is welcome even in the safety of our own home, so that our brain feels secure enough to put our body into the almost paralyzed state associated with REM and deep sleep.

I've read various so-called psychological studies pontificating on what your sleeping position says about your personality, but the only thing that adopting my recommended sleeping position says about you is that you are taking your mental and physical recovery seriously.

The Mattress Checkup

You can now perform the mattress checkup, which is as effective with your existing mattress as it is when you are trying out a new one. This is precisely what our young couple at the start of the chapter should have been doing in the mattress store.

A partner or friend is useful to have around to do the checkup, but you could use the camera on your phone. At home, stand with a good, upright posture and your arms gently folded. Bend your knees—effectively do a shallow squat—into a comfortable and balanced position. This is your standing fetal position.

Adopt this position on the floor, lying on your non-dominant side, and hold this posture for a little while. Your partner or friend will acknowledge the gap between your head and the floor, or you can take a selfie on your camera to see it, and you'll certainly feel it in your neck (pillows would traditionally fill this gap). As you lie there, with your posture aligned and the pressure building on your shoulder and hip on the unforgiving surface, you'll feel the urge to move and adjust, which commonly happens to us during sleep—particularly on surfaces that are too firm—or the surface will simply aggravate sensitive muscles and joints. Now, you could sleep here on the floor (and you'd probably end up lying on your stomach), but you are sacrificing the quality of recovery.

You should then adopt this position on the mattress you're checking. If it's your mattress at home, strip the bed, including the pillows, so it's just the bare mattress; in a mattress store, you'll often be testing on a bare mattress, but go ahead and pull the sheets back if not. Once you're settled in position, again get a friend or partner—or take a selfie—to judge the gap between your head and the surface.

If there is a clear gap of two and a half inches—about the width of two hands flat on top of one another—or more between your head and the mattress when your head, neck, and vertebrae are in alignment, with your head needing to drop

The Fetal Position on a Correctly Profiled Surface

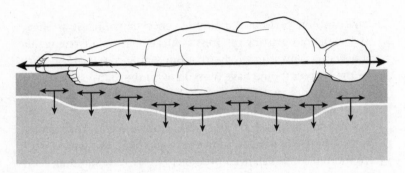

toward the surface, as it did on the floor, then the mattress is too firm. It will offer you little in the way of comfort and postural alignment. If your hip is dropping into the mattress and out of alignment, and your head is being raised up by the mattress, then it is too soft. The correctly profiled surface should easily accept your body shape and weight, distributing your weight evenly and giving you a straight postural line, like the diagram on this page.

If you are trying a mattress in a store and it is not doing this for you, move along. No matter what it is made of or what it cost, if your mattress at home isn't doing this, it's time to think about replacing it. But don't despair if you can't afford to—there are less expensive measures that can be taken to compensate for it.

The right mattress pad or topper will sit on top and provide an extension to your mattress that will be able to better provide the body profile requirements you need when you sleep. A pillow-top pad, which is essentially a mattress-size body pillow, can be added to improve the comfort and protect sensitive muscles and joints. You could use a spare comforter to achieve similar results, with your bedsheet on top.

However, many of us are already compensating for the wrong mattress every night with the use of something that, as the diagram suggests, we shouldn't really need.

Pillow Talk

If you go shoe shopping, you find the footwear you like and ask for it in your correct size. If the shop doesn't have it, you're left with a choice. You can't really contemplate going smaller, because you'll be in pain when you walk, but you can go a size bigger if you're willing to add insoles.

A pillow is an insole for a mattress that does not fit. We use them to fill that gap between the head and the surface when the mattress is too firm, and when the mattress is too soft, they push our head even further out of alignment and can cause postural problems. If you are sleeping on two or even more pillows, then either you've got a very firm mattress or you're storing up trouble for yourself.

You can buy memory-foam pillows, feather pillows, cheapo polyester-fill pillows, anti-snoring pillows, and even that label beloved of the bed industry, orthopedic pillows. Some come in wonderfully exotic fabrics and fillings (Siberian goose down!), others in the most basic of man-made fibers, but they all look pretty much the same with a pillowcase on them. It doesn't matter what their manufacturers claim of them or how much they cost, they're all doing the same job—compensating for your mattress.

If we have the right sleeping surface, a pillow is on the verge of being entirely superfluous. But they're a difficult habit to kick. We like pillows—we're used to them. We like to hold on to them in the night. We like to rearrange them and fluff them up before we get into bed, and we love to wrestle with them and pound them into submission when we're struggling to sleep. So a *single* shallow pillow for comfort will be just fine for you, as on the correctly profiled mattress it will compress to fit. And better a bargain-basement polyester pillow that fits the profile than an expensive "orthopedic" neck brace of a pillow that is going to cause you problems.

Supersize Me

The young couple made many mistakes when they chose a mattress, but they made perhaps their biggest before they even set foot in the store—when they decided to buy a queen-size bed.

For most of us as children, our first beds are a standard single or twin bed, so called because they were often marketed as a pair. A twin is 38 inches (a little more than three feet) by 75 inches (six feet three inches). We might keep a twin throughout adolescence and early adulthood, but usually when we leave home we upgrade to a full-size bed.

A full or double bed is 53 inches wide (four feet five inches). Meanwhile, a queen-size mattress is 60 inches (five feet) wide. You don't have to be a mathematician to figure out that there's nothing "double" about either of them. If you've spent most of your life up to a certain age with a twin bed's worth of space, what's going to happen when you add an extra person but only around 50 percent more space? Do you think it's likely to maintain the quality of your sleep?

Despite what their labeling claims, bed retailers only sell one genuine "double" bed. It's called a king—so branded to make it sound like a suitably decadent purchase—and it measures in at 76 inches (six feet four inches) wide, exactly double the width of a twin bed. If you're serious about sleep, and you're serious about your relationship, and you have the room for it, this is the *minimum* size of mattress you should be considering. A king is two single-size sleeping spaces side by side; a so-called double is really a bed for one person.

If you do have space for a king but it means your bedside tables would have to go, set them free. This is more important. If your bed frame is the problem and you can't afford to replace it, set that free too and put the new mattress on the floor. The young couple spent 50 percent of their original budget on a frame. Most sources will recommend spending more on the mattress than the frame, but you could just as easily spend 100 percent on the mattress. I don't even make bed frames; I only produce sleeping surfaces. The frame is a largely decorative choice, to make the bedroom look good. As long as it's a firm and level surface for the mattress to rest on, it doesn't matter what it is. You could use wooden pallets, which are a fashionable, industrial-chic, and low-cost choice, or the floor. Many athletes actually prefer sleeping in their sleep kit on the floor, as it's cooler there (heat rises).

The less room we have in bed, the more we're likely to disturb a partner's sleep. A stray leg or arm touching you in the night, a partner turning over and fussing with their pillow right next to you, a partner *breathing* on you up close—they can pull you out of a cycle and stop you from getting down to the deep sleep your mind and body deserve.

Building a Sleep Kit

In 2009, Shane Sutton, the head coach of British Cycling at the time, put me in touch with Matt Parker, the head of marginal gains. The academic and clinical expertise on sleep they had looked into had proven too intrusive and impractical to use, so I worked very closely with Matt, drawing upon the techniques and interventions I'd established over the years, to see where recovery gains could be unlocked. I then presented our redefined approach to mental and physical recovery to the performance director, Dave Brailsford, and his extensive team of the best coaches and sports science professionals from across the globe. The reaction was simple: "This could really make a difference."

It was an exciting time to get involved in cycling. Sky's significant investment in British Cycling—the country's governing body—allowed them to launch a professional team, signing up some of the best riders, including Bradley Wiggins, with the ambition of putting a British rider at the top of the podium at the Tour de France.

To this end, the team was addressing everything from the obvious things like the bikes, fitness, and tactics to the less overt

such as psychology, avoiding viruses (there's no point in showing up at the grueling Tour de France with a nagging cough),
and, of course, sleep. All of this was part of their "aggregation of
marginal gains" approach, in which they sought to take every
individual component involved in the sport and better it, even
by just 1 percent, so that when it all came together the improvement could be significant.

I laid out the Key Sleep Recovery Indicators and showed not
just the riders but every member of the staff the importance of
sleeping in cycles, the necessity of using recovery breaks, and
how to maintain their environment at home, educating them
in the R90 program. But I knew that I could have more of an
impact.

The key to the approach in other fields was consistency. The
riders were on the same nutritional plan all the time, riding the
same bike, and wearing the same gear—but they were sleeping
in a different hotel room, on a different bed, every night when
they were riding on a tour event. So I designed and produced
the R90 sleep kit for the riders to enable them to sleep on the
same custom-designed surface every night.

The sleep kit is basically a portable single-size bed. It is
composed of two or three layers, depending on the rider, of
viscoelastic memory foam—essentially two or three mattress
toppers—with a pillow-top pad on top. This is wrapped in a removable machine-washable outer cover, combined with a shallow pillow and combination comforter and bedsheets. All of
this is housed within a specially designed backpack, so it can be
folded in half, zipped up, and carried out in a matter of seconds.
To use it again, simply carry it into the room, unzip it, and put
it wherever you need it—either on the bed base (we'd move the
existing mattress out of the way) or right on the floor. It's ready
to use.

For the riders, it was a revelation. It meant that they could
have their sleep kits at home and become used to sleeping on
them in the way I'd shown them, and then we would load up
the Sky bus with everyone's kits. So when the riders retired to

their rooms after a hard day in the saddle, they would know what was waiting for them: the support staff had already been in and laid down their sleep kits. It was familiar to them, because they'd been sleeping on it for weeks. When they left in the morning, the staff went back in to zip them up and take them out—and the riders knew that they'd be sleeping on exactly the same surface the following night. Yes, there were some strange looks from the other teams as Sky arrived at each hotel and started bringing in a kit for every rider. It wasn't just for the riders either—the staff on the team bus had their own sleep kits. It was a top-down approach, looking for the marginal gains in everyone's role.

On his Tour de France–winning campaign in 2012, Bradley Wiggins's mattress was basically a couple of pieces of foam. At the 2012 London Olympics, cyclist Chris Hoy would ignore the bed and sleep on the floor of his five-star-hotel room on his own sleep kit, correctly profiled for his very different body shape, of course. When he traveled to the Olympic Village in Stratford, London, to compete, winning two gold medals in the process, he did so in a helicopter with his sleep kit loaded in there with him.

These athletes, just like their teammates, were putting their bodies on the line, day after day, and required the very best in terms of mental and physical recovery—and if they didn't need a heavy multi-thousand-coil mattress like our young couple bought, why would you?

Building Your Sleep Kit

While Team Sky is able to buy a custom-made product for each cyclist, tailored to their exact measurements, they aren't the only people I provide sleep kits for. I also work with athletes who don't have any funding from their national sport association and so have to live within more modest means. This includes teenage BMX riders with an eye on the Olympics in 2020 whose only source of funding is their parents, and enthusiastic amateur cyclists who want the best in recovery at a reasonable price point. It has to be affordable for these people too.

If you follow the principles that guide the professional athletes, you can create your own custom sleep kit. You won't be carrying it around the world, of course—it will be a domestic version, ideally king-size, with components sourced from wherever you choose, according to your budget, to give you the very best chance of making the most of your nocturnal cycles.

Piece by Piece

Some retailers claim you should change your mattress every seven years; some manufacturers claim theirs will last you ten years. This is the kind of logic that leads our young couple to spend $1,500 on a mattress, thinking that it works out to only $150 a year. But I would rather see you spend $150 on your sleeping surface every year, or $300 every couple of years, for ten years than spend the whole $1,500 at once. When I was sales and marketing director of the Slumberland Group and chairman of the UK Sleep Council, I was part of an industry initiative to encourage sleepers to change their beds more often. The average bed's life span was more like twenty-plus years, so manufacturers and retailers got together to promote a change at ten years.

(Even today, the message is unclear, because if we are asked to change our beds every seven to ten years, why do we have ten-year or lifetime guarantees? It's all about reassuring you that the "right way" to buy a mattress is to spend every penny in your budget.)

Think about what you get up to on your mattress. You have sex on it. You sweat all over it during the hot summer months. You might have the occasional takeout dinner on it when you're enjoying a lazy day, or eat breakfast in bed on the weekend. If you have children, they might jump in and make all kinds of messes. Some people even let their pets on their bed. With all those bodily fluids, hair, and dead skin cells only a sheet's width away from it, why would you want to hold on to a mattress for ten years? To get sentimental about the stains?

It's not just the superficial damage. Mattresses degrade over time. The fresh-out-of-the-box springy surface you invested in will inevitably head south with age. The properties will deteriorate after around eight hours per night of your (and your partner's, if you have one) body weight on top of them. Dust mites, which we'll come to shortly, are increasingly likely to have set up camp.

Instead of this every-ten-years approach, you could build your sleep kit piece by piece. Start with your core surface. This could be your existing mattress, or you could buy one that better fits your (and your partner's) profile, which might only cost $200 or $300, and add layers to that (2–3 inches deep is fine for extra layers), building it up. If your existing mattress isn't correctly profiled, these layers will improve it at a fraction of the cost of replacing the mattress. If you have a well-profiled mattress, another layer could still improve upon it and offer you even better comfort.

Add a pillow-top pad to go on top of the core surface. The sleep kits I make have a mattress cover that can be removed and washed, so you can get rid of any unwanted stains, unlike the stitched-up permanent covers of most commercially available products. Add this feature, or at least a mattress protector, to your own kit.

You have the potential to build your own, tailored-to-you sleeping surface, sourcing the elements from wherever you choose so long as they fit your profile. If you build it incrementally, you will feel less hesitation about replacing sections of it in a few years rather than every ten because it hasn't cost you $1,500. The stains and natural degrading of materials we talked about earlier aren't as important, because they are simply affecting the layers on top, which will be replaced more regularly.

I send portable sleep kits and foam mattress toppers all over the world for events. The high-grade memory foam I use can be rolled up and packed so that shipping costs are kept down. Once the athlete has used it, they might even decide not to bring it home with them afterward. It's not quite a disposable item, but compared to a $1,500 slab, it certainly feels more like it. The athlete might give it to charity or to a local sports academy if it isn't coming home with them, or it can travel on with them.

Bedding

Your sleep kit covers should ideally be hypoallergenic; in fact, all your bedding should, whether you suffer from allergies or not.

Dust mites live in carpets, clothing, and bedding; they love humid environments and feast on your dead skin flakes. It isn't the mites themselves that trigger allergic reactions, it's their droppings. In the wrong kind of environment, you could be lying down to sleep in a cloud of their fecal particles.

People in sports can tend toward mouth-breathing, particularly when they're competing and they're trying to suck in as much oxygen as possible. Allergens can affect breathing during the night, making it difficult to breathe through the nose, resulting in the mouth-breathing complications—snoring, sleep apnea, dry mouth—that can potentially pull someone out of a sleep cycle. If you are sleeping in hypoallergenic bedding (mattress, mattress cover, sheets, comforter, duvet cover, pillow, pillowcase), it's another marginal gain.

The bedding in your sleep kit also needs to be breathable, so that you don't experience any unwelcome changes in temperature. We need to be cool under the covers, and if it gets too stuffy and warm under there, it will interfere with our sleep. The bedding I use is designed with nanotechnology and uses microfibers a fraction of the diameter of a human hair, the pillow uses this material too in order to keep your head cool, and the comforters are lightweight and breathable, while providing the requisite tog rating (a level of thermal insulation—if you buy a comforter in Britain, it will be labeled with its tog rating, but in the United States you might see this only on bedding for babies and toddlers). I do recommend a duvet cover, the protective removable cover for your warm comforter, rather than a comforter alone. That way, you can remove and wash the cover. When it's particularly warm, just use the duvet cover on its own. This gives you more options to control your body temperature as the seasons change. Not all hotel temperatures are the same, so if a rider comes down and says it's a little warm in his room, we can change the comforter to compensate.

The bed linens are all white, which is clean and neutral. The blanket or comforter itself is lightweight enough to be machine washable, which means that it will perform more efficiently. Take this approach to your home kit, as there's no excuse for the kind of dirty, stained old bedding that many people own.

Cleanliness, in fact, is of major benefit when it comes to bedding. It took me some time to work up the courage to share one of my ideas for the portable sleep kits with Matt Parker and the coaches at British Cycling: ensuring that the riders had fresh bed linens every single night. There's nothing particularly scientific behind the idea. I just know that when I have fresh sheets on my bed, I look forward to getting into it. It's clean, it's cool, it's an incredibly welcoming environment—I climb in and immediately feel relaxed, so I can just switch off and drift away immediately in it, enjoying a refreshing night's sleep. So why not every night? Thankfully, Matt got it right away—even if it did mean commandeering the washing machines on the team bus, which were used to wash the riders' cycling gear. Because of that constraint the bedding had to be quick-drying, which ruled out Egyptian cotton, but because ours was made from hypoallergenic microfiber, drying time wasn't a problem. It could be washed in cold water and dried in minutes, and at the end of a long day in the mountains the riders would have fresh bed linens. It's the little things sometimes.

This is a very easy gain to make in your own life. Stripping the bed, washing the sheets, and remaking the bed every day is obviously not an appealing prospect for anyone, but how often do you wash your sheets? If it's every two weeks, why not try taking it down to every week? Simply double up on what you already do and you'll enjoy the benefits. You'll get to enjoy fresh bedding just a little bit more often, and your bed will become a more consistently inviting place. Changing bed linens is also a great pre-sleep routine.

As the R90 sleep kit is composed of man-made materials, it might leave the more environmentally minded reader a little uncomfortable when they're considering their home kit. The simple fact is that in sports we're interested in gold medals and podium finishes first, and the environment second. That's not to say we're not interested in the environment away from the competitive arena—I take all sorts of measures to reduce my environmental footprint, and the future for sleep-science technology will keep the fate of our vulnerable planet very much in mind, with things like inflatable mattresses and layers, and recovery suits that only require a sheet to control our body temperature.

For now, man-made materials are simply better. Nanotechnology can make the fibers a fraction of the size of any naturally occurring product, so breathability and speed to dry can't be beaten. If you're uncomfortable about this, or if you simply can't do without your Egyptian cotton, then go for a thread count of around 300 in your own sleep kit, which will offer you the best natural breathability. And look at changing your pillows and blankets more regularly if you haven't gone for the hypoallergenic options. Just like the mattress, an inexpensive pillow correctly profiled and regularly replaced is better than an expensive wrong one you plan on getting several years out of.

Turning In

It's important to be realistic about what a product in isolation is going to do for you. But following these guidelines to build your own home sleep kit alongside the rest of the R90 program, when you are ticking all the right boxes around your sleep, will revolutionize your recovery.

The effect the portable sleep kits had on the Team Sky riders on the Grand Tours was quite dramatic. Whereas before you would catch the riders milling around and putting off going to bed, maybe having a massage or talking tactics, after the introduction of the sleep kits they would get everything sorted out and then head straight to their rooms. They had the confidence to know that after two hundred kilometers in the mountains, with their bodies spent, they could go upstairs, climb into their sleep kit in the fetal position, breathe softly through their nose, and drift away into their cycles of sleep.

If you get your own home sleep kit right, you can know this confidence too. No more walking into this process blind, like the young couple at the start of the chapter. No more tossing and turning to get yourself comfortable. No more shifting on to your front, your back, and then your side. You will know with absolute certainty that you can just get into bed in the fetal position on your non-dominant side, close your eyes, breathe through your nose, and then . . . just drift away.

THE SLEEP KIT:
SEVEN STEPS TO SLEEP SMARTER

1. Learn to sleep in the fetal position, on your non-dominant side (left-handed people sleep on their right, right-handers on their left).

2. Do the mattress checkup and know what your correctly profiled surface feels like. Do the same for your sleeping partner.

3. Take an incremental approach: spend $500 twice over seven years on your sleeping surface rather than $1,000 all at once. Think about layers that can be washed and replaced regularly.

4. Use hypoallergenic and breathable bedding, whether you have allergies or not, to keep out potential impediments to sleep and regulate your temperature.

5. Size matters—buy as big as you can. A king mattress is the minimum size a couple should contemplate (space permitting); a full-size or "double" bed is a bed for one person.

6. Don't buy blind! Engage with the salesperson's knowledge to help define what is available, but use what you have learned in this chapter when it comes to making the final choice.

7. Remember the mattress-to-bed-frame ratio of importance: the mattress can be as much as 100 percent of your budget because the bed frame is effectively a decorative item.

SEVEN

Recovery Room

The Sleeping Environment

When a leading NFL team asks me to come in and talk to the team about sleep, and then their star player—let's call him Rod—asks me to come to his home and have a look at his sleeping environment there, I am happy to help. Who could say no to an offer like that?

Rod's is a not untypical sports star's mansion: enough security to make Fort Knox blush, a sports car in the driveway, a vast entryway, many rooms stocked by interior designers with custom furniture and investment art, the latest flat-screen televisions and audio equipment in every room, and futuristic gadgets everywhere. It might be easy for the casual observer to pass judgment, but my view is that the top professional athletes work hard and have to deal with a lot of intrusion and pressure, so why shouldn't they enjoy spending the money they earn?

I cut straight to the chase and ask Rod to show me his bedroom. Football players talk about the sanctity of the locker room, so what does that make the bedroom? The people who allow me in are effectively asking me to judge the environment in which they spend their most vulnerable time (asleep) and usually their most intimate time (with their partners).

Rod's housekeeper has obviously made a visit recently. No one wants to make a bad impression—with, say, underwear on the floor and the bed unmade—so I never see the environment *exactly* as it is from day to day, but I see more than enough to make an assessment.

I immediately notice the huge wide-screen television at the foot of the bed. With the click of a button, it will slide out and rise to viewing level, along with some serious-looking surround-sound speakers, for the full cinematic experience in bed. "You should see *Fast and Furious* on this thing," Rod says, laughing.

There is a videogame console in there too, and the rest of the room is similarly decked out in high-tech gadgetry. There are smartphone docks and laptops and tablets everywhere, and an impressive array of standby lights illuminating the room. There is a filtered water dispenser by the bed, I note, and as for the bed itself, it's big enough—a custom size that would dwarf even a California king—for Rod and his wife, who is a model, a definite ectomorph to Rod's classic mesomorph profile. I check the mattress, an expensive spring-packed slab filled with horse-hair, and the Siberian goose-down comforter—all of which will roast them nicely over the course of a night.

Speaking of which, it's warm in the room, so I glance at the temperature on the electronic control on the wall. It's 75 degrees. "Is it always set to this?" I ask.

"Oh, yes," says Rod. "My wife likes it nice and toasty in here at night."

There is a mountain of plump pillows at the head of the bed. The remote-controlled blinds in the windows look fancy, but a little light leaks in when they're closed. The walls seem solid enough and, with the double-paned windows closed, there is an impressive layer of sound insulation. I check the doors both to the bedroom and the en suite bathroom, and note the slivers of light that leak in under them.

I'm taking in the fashionable color scheme and the huge pieces of bright, eye-catching art adorning the walls, along with a few framed jerseys, when Rod's wife pops her head in the door. "Can I get you a drink?" she asks. Looking around the rest of the house—getting a better feel for the individual's lifestyle outside the bedroom—is always a good idea, but it's not always an easy thing to ask without sounding nosy. An open invitation is always welcome, of course.

I follow the couple out of the bedroom down to the space-age kitchen, fitted out with every appliance imaginable—including a top-of-the-line single-serve coffee and espresso machine. "That's a beauty," I say.

"I need my red-eye in the morning before I head to practice," says Rod. "Only way to get through the day. Want one?" I think about the caffeine supplements and gum he will consume in addition to this.

"Just a regular coffee for me, please, Rod."

The Sanctuary

Rod is not at all unusual among football players—and, not just to pick on those who play the sport at the highest level, he's not unusual among people generally.

While an NFL star might have all the money in the world to spend on sabotaging their sleep in a bedroom like that, the truth is that excess isn't the cause of it. I can just as easily go to an Olympic athlete's bedroom and see them handicap their sleep by more modest means: the standby light on the television; the smartphone charger plugged into the socket by the bed; the flimsy, transparent blinds; the bottle of water on the bedside table; the bookshelf stacked with thrillers and horror classics.

You might wonder how some of these factors will affect sleep, but if we look at your bedroom in comparison to our island in Chapter 1, with the two of us sitting by the fire, we can see how far things have moved away from our sleep ideal.

The bedroom once did what its name promised: there would be a bed, some furniture such as a wardrobe and dresser, a bedside table, and maybe a vanity table or desk. Children would have their toys in there, and books would feature in some bedrooms; alarm clocks and lamps too, of course. Technology changed things, first with televisions in the bedroom, and to-day with the multitude of devices that allow us to watch movies, listen to music, interact on social media, and play video games from the comfort of our bed. The bedroom has effectively become an extra living space instead of a room for sleep.

For some people this is simply a fact of life. Adolescents have always made their bedroom a parent-free sanctuary in which to indulge their solo pursuits (and, we hope, do their homework). College students in residence halls and shared houses have to make do with a single room in which to study, sleep, and have some personal downtime. In fact, it makes financial sense for many people in their twenties and even their thirties to continue living with roommates as they set out on their careers. But what we're seeing now is this trend continuing even with people into their forties and beyond, who have good incomes and careers, because prices in both the buying and rental markets, particularly in metropolitan areas like New York, San Francisco, and London, are spiraling out of control.

Like the marginal-gains approach, we need to look toward stripping away as many of the potential obstacles as possible as we head toward a sleep state. And if we can't strip them away—Rod is not in a hurry to give up watching *Fast and Furious* in bed—then we need to at least learn to control their impact.

We have already covered the most important item in the bedroom, the sleep kit, but getting that right isn't going to do you any good at all if the environment it's in is all wrong. Our bedrooms must become a sleep sanctuary—a mental and physical recovery room—if we're to get the maximum benefit from the R90 program.

Cut the Crap

When I traveled with England's soccer team to the Euro 2004 Championships in Portugal, I did so knowing that I could have an impact on their hotel rooms far beyond what I could achieve in their homes.

The team would be staying at the same hotel for the whole tournament, so there would be no moving around—no planning for and adjusting to a new environment every night, as I would need to do a few years later with the cycling team. This was a great opportunity to have a controlled, consistent environment for the players' recovery, I thought. The manager, Sven-Göran Eriksson, and Leif Sward, the doctor, agreed, so I went out to Lisbon in advance to set things up.

We brought in our own "beds," the media gleefully reported (in fact, they were an early incarnation of my sleep kit—custom-made viscoelastic memory foam mattress toppers, which weren't as easily available then as they are today), and used the hotel rooms as a blank canvas on which we could paint the perfect sleeping environment for the players.

Of course, while I took care of the rooms themselves, the Football Association (FA) went to much greater lengths to protect the privacy of those sleeping in them. That particular English squad was a star-studded bunch, with the likes of David Beckham and Steven Gerrard in the ranks, both of whom would go on to one day play for the LA Galaxy, and Sven was a tabloid draw too. So the FA had thirty-foot-tall fir trees brought in and planted around the perimeter to stop the paparazzi from getting any pictures.

Alongside the new beds and huge trees, there were slot machines, chefs, and all sorts of food for specific dietary requirements—I'd never seen anything like it, and neither had the hotel staff. But there was a real buzz about the place. That squad of players, as well as being star-studded, had a genuine chance of doing well at the tournament. Being able to control their sleeping environment was a real marginal gain to be made.

Today, soccer organizations take this idea seriously. At Real Madrid, each of the players has a luxury apartment available at their training facility. These rooms can only be unlocked by the individual player's fingerprint and are equipped with high-end bathrooms, beds, and televisions. Manchester City adopted a similar approach with their new £200 million training complex that included rooms for the players. They don't quite match the Real Madrid accommodations in terms of luxury, but as I hope I've made clear so far, it's not just about five-star facilities when it comes to recovery. Dr. Sam Erith, head of sports science for Manchester United, brought me in to consult on recovery at this state-of-the-art complex, and the rooms have all the ingredients to allow the players to get the maximum rewards from their time spent in them.

These rooms serve many benefits, allowing the players to rest between training sessions for one, but mainly in being able to control the players' sleeping environment before a home game (or an away game, if they're playing a nearby club such as local rivals Manchester United) and minimize their disruption on the day of the game. Manchester City players will spend the night before the match at the training-facility accommodation, so when they get up, they're all there, ready to have breakfast and prepare for the game. They don't have to travel, there's no danger of any complications making them late. As it's not a hotel room, there's no need to worry about the effect the hotel staff or guests might have on the environment: it's all in the club's control.

They're useful after an evening home game too. It means that when the match finishes, by the time the player has attended to his media obligations, showered and changed, and consulted with the staff as needed—be that a word with his manager or a rubdown from the masseur—he's not going to have to drive home late at night tired and staring down the barrel of fewer sleep cycles that night. He can just head straight to his room at the training facility, go through his pre-sleep routine, and recover there.

We can emulate the Manchester City and Real Madrid experience in our own homes. While the fingerprint technology is likely to be beyond most of us, we can at least start with our own blank canvas. This means taking everything out of your current bedroom. You could literally do this if you felt so committed, but doing it in your head works just as well.

The Empty Shell

This empty room is no longer a bedroom, nor is it an extension of your living space. Starting here, it is your mental and physical *recovery room*.

My first piece of advice would be to paint it white and put nothing back on the walls. We don't want any potential stimulus in the room that a loud color scheme or pictures on the walls might provide, just a very simple, clean, and neutral decor.

Then we look at controlling one of the key bedroom prompts for our circadian rhythms—light—with curtains or blinds. We produce melatonin in darkness, so we need our recovery rooms to be free of ambient light such as streetlights. Total blackout is the most effective method, but an eye mask, which can cause discomfort and interfere with your sleep, is not ideal. If your curtains or blinds leak light around the edges, or they are flimsy and transparent, replacing them would be a sensible option. Blackout roller blinds can be bought relatively inexpensively, and there are even cheaper alternatives: you could tape the curtains closed or use Velcro fasteners to attach easily removable blackout material to the windows at night. On the Grand Tours, as I've mentioned, we would sometimes tape black trash bags to the windows, as they could easily be taken down in the morning.

We need daylight in the morning, of course, so once you wake up at your constant time, it's essential to get the blinds or curtains open immediately and flick that internal switch to get you producing serotonin. If light is leaking in during the summer months, you are likely to find that you're waking up with it at 5 a.m. instead of your constant wake time of 7 a.m. Blackout allows you to control this.

Temperature Control

Temperature is, after the move from light to dark, the next most important factor to get right so that we can best work with our circadian rhythms and fall into a sleep state. Our bodies want to move into a cooler (but not cold) environment, just as we did around our fire in Chapter 1, so keeping the room at an optimal 60 to 65 degrees Fahrenheit will allow this natural process to occur. Of course, we all have different sensitivities to temperature—for some, 65 degrees might sound a little *too* close to sleeping outside with nature—so find a temperature that works for you (and your partner) that is cooler than the environment in the rest of the house. If you have a sophisticated heating system, the bedroom thermostat can be set accordingly, but for the rest of us it can be as simple as opening the window an hour before going to bed or turning off the radiator while the heating is on in the rest of the house. Whatever the temperature is, warm to cool is the mantra.

Importing the Essentials

The first thing we put back into the recovery room is, of course, your sleep kit. This, along with an alarm clock of some description, which we'll come to shortly, is the only genuinely essential piece that you need back in this room. Anything else is unnecessary from the point of view of recovery.

If you're able to, put your clothes and your dresser or wardrobe—anything that isn't essential for sleep—elsewhere. However, that's just not realistic for most of us, and these items will have to come back into the room. What constitutes "essential" will be different for all of us too. For a student living in a dorm room, it will mean the return of their desk and workspace, although work is an activity better kept out of the recovery room if you have the option.

If you work from home and have your desk in the bedroom, try to work at the kitchen table or out of the room if possible, so your mind doesn't make an association between the recovery room and work. If you have bookshelves in your room stacked with thrillers and horror books, think about the stimulus this gives your mind when you look at them before sleep. They are not calm and relaxing associations for your mind to make.

A bottle of water may seem like a fairly standard and innocuous item to bring into the room at night, but why do you need it? If you wake with a dry mouth during the night, it's likely to be because you're breathing through your mouth rather than your nose, and if you get up during the night to go to the bathroom, it's possible that you have been overhydrating in the lead-up to sleep. Putting a bottle of water by your bedside plants the idea of drinking it in your mind.

The only thing you want your mind to associate this room with is sleep.

Tech Attack

Your recovery room needs an alarm clock—ideally a dawn simulator—that isn't your phone. No other technology is necessary.

A dawn simulator will wake you up gradually with artificial daylight, starting thirty minutes before your alarm time. These devices are not just for those suffering from seasonal affective disorder (SAD) but for anyone who wants to replicate the rising of the sun so that they wake more naturally. Dawn simulators can improve alertness, cognitive and physical performance, mood, and well-being.[1] In winter, they can be the difference between getting straight out of your sleep kit and hitting the snooze button. And in a blacked-out room they are the most effective way to get you up so you can then open the blinds and let natural light in.

This technology doesn't have to be expensive—a basic model will do, provided it's from a reputable brand such as Philips or Lumie. And if you can't swing that, use a standard alarm clock, provided you can turn off the illumination on the display so the light doesn't bother you at night. (If you choose an analog option, make sure it doesn't produce a ticking noise that could keep you awake.)

The light here is key. There's no point blocking out all the artificial light from outside if you're going to fill your room up with it. As soon as you start bringing televisions and electronic devices back into the bedroom, you're bringing in light sources. Your pre-sleep routine involves paring back on technology as you approach the time to go into a sleep state, but if you really can't avoid watching television, using your laptop, or playing on your game console in bed, please just do one thing for your recovery when you've finished: turn the devices off properly, instead of hitting standby. The standby light is like a laser penetrating all the way through to your pineal gland and interfering with your melatonin production.

The most damaging piece of technology at night, however, is the smartphone. According to Ofcom, the communications regulator in the United Kingdom, four in ten smartphone users reported using their phones after the devices had woken them in bed during the night.[2] Furthermore, even if they have been silenced, the artificial light they emit is another problem. If you can't stop yourself from using your phone as part of your pre-sleep routine, try to build toward it with the tech breaks we talked about in Chapter 5. At the very least, you can keep it out of your way while you are asleep: in another room, in a drawer, or turned off completely. What could you be missing out on? Even the most avid social media user can't do it in their sleep.

Keep It Clean!

Professional cyclists are a sensitive bunch—sensitive to their environment, that is. They have to be, given how damaging picking up an unwanted bug could be to their performance. Before they arrived at their hotel every night we would enter the rooms and put a HEPA (high-efficiency particulate air) filter in to remove unwanted airborne particles, and then we would use a hand vacuum and antibacterial cleaning products to wipe all the surfaces down, being sure to attend to the hidden corners where the hotel cleaners might not have reached. As I've said before, it's a glamorous world on tour.

While you don't need to go to this level of obsessive cleanliness, keeping your recovery room clean is a worthwhile pursuit. Who doesn't want to breathe clean air? There is the subconscious reassurance, much like fresh sheets provide, that you are moving into a clean environment to sleep. Dust mites live in carpets as well as bedding, so if you are an allergy sufferer, a HEPA filter that emits no sound or light would be a good investment to help you get down through the stages to deep sleep every night.

A clutter-free environment is also preferable. "If a cluttered desk is the sign of a cluttered mind, then what is an empty desk?" goes the saying, but an empty mind, having downloaded your thoughts in your pre-sleep routine, is a welcome sign before we enter sleep. Clothes all over the floor and items piling up on the surfaces can provide stimulus to the mind (although for some people, clutter-free means having clothes piled up in the *right* places on the floor).

Noise Control

Noise is a big factor in waking us from light sleep. If your name is called or a door is slammed loud enough when you are in this stage, you will wake up. Adequate soundproofing such as double-paned windows is great to keep out external noise, but those of us living in rented accommodations are usually stuck with what we've got. Unluckier still are those who live in houses and apartments where the soundproofing is woefully inadequate between floors and walls (and you can hear the neighbors get up to all sorts of things at night). Soundproofing in such instances is expensive, so earplugs provide the answer for many people. They can be effective up to a point, but the discomfort they can cause might disturb sleep.

There can be helpful noise too. In his 2006 autobiography, English soccer star Wayne Rooney admits to needing the sound of a vacuum cleaner or hair dryer to fall asleep to. This isn't as unusual as it might sound—many people find the hum of an air conditioner or the dull rumble of traffic (if they live near a road) just as necessary. This sound functions as a kind of "white noise," which masks the peaks and troughs of background noise that might otherwise disturb them from light sleep. You can download white noise to use in the bedroom, as a vacuum cleaner or hairdryer manufacturer is unlikely to recommend leaving one of their products on unattended all night.

Security

Perhaps the most important role our recovery room should play—even more so than its engineering for our light-dark and temperature cycles—is in providing us with a feeling of security. We need to feel safe and relaxed in our recovery room so that we can fall asleep easily and rest properly. We are going into our most vulnerable state, and reducing any fear or anxiety surrounding this is paramount.

This idea of security can come in many forms. It could mean locking all the doors and windows in your home as part of your pre-sleep routine; it could be something more personal, such as having a picture of loved ones by your sleep kit or a favorite comfort blanket in there with you. Whatever it is that you need to give you that feeling of security, so that your mind is able to switch off from a state of alert and relax into your designated cycles of sleep, is a welcome addition to the room. We take this approach with elite athletes. If a performer needs his or her favorite teddy bear to sleep, it comes with us. Anything to produce the safest and most secure environment for them to go into a sleep state.

RECOVERY ROOM:
SEVEN STEPS TO SLEEP SMARTER

1. Your bedroom should not be an extension of your living space, if possible. Rename it your mental and physical recovery room.

2. Empty your room (if only in your head) and bring back only the items necessary for rest, recovery, and relaxation.

3. Black out your room so that external light does not interfere with your sleep.

4. Make your room a cooler (but not cold) environment compared to the rest of the home.

5. Feel safe and secure in your room—a favorite stuffed animal, a picture of loved ones, or double-checking that the doors and windows are locked can all help.

6. Have a neutral decor, keep it clean, and avoid anything that is likely to stimulate the mind (bright pictures or books with which you make strong personal connections).

7. Control tech use in your room. Turn standby lights off at night, and have your phone either out of the room or at least out of sight (and silenced).

PART TWO

R90 in Action

EIGHT

A Head Start

Using Your R90 Recovery Program

It's March 2016, and thirty full sleep kits boxed up in individual packages a fraction of the size of an upholstered mattress are on a boat, traveling across the Atlantic Ocean to Rio for the Olympic Games. The athletes won't actually be competing until August, but this being one of the biggest sporting events on the planet, the levels of security and bureaucracy are sky high: every item heading into the Olympic Village has to be approved and accounted for. There's no point turning up with a brand-new track bike if you haven't had it pre-approved.

We've been busy for twelve months prior to this. The organization on the ground in Rio has been, frankly, something of a mess, and we haven't been able to get much in the way of information. But we now know what the beds in the athletes' accommodations will be: single beds, with an extending twelve-inch piece for the taller athletes; the mattresses, rock hard. We know that it will be very hot out there, and we've discovered that the rooms will not come with air conditioners as standard. That has now been rectified with portable units.

The sailors have been out in August, the year before, and they've spoken of sailing in waters polluted beyond belief. But no matter how much of a mess things appear in the run-up to an Olympics, they always seem to work out in the end, and Rio will be no different.

There are other factors at play: drug scandals, political crises in the governing bodies, and Zika virus worries. We can't control these. We simply work on the elements we can control, and improving the sleeping environment is my part in this. We can't control the other teams either, and the kind of planning they might have under way. But our months of work in every aspect of our preparation mean that we have done everything possible that we can to give ourselves a head start.

Recovery Schedule

Through combining the seven Key Sleep Recovery Indicators together to form the R90 program, we can get a head start too. Our days no longer consist of periods of time at work, at home, and at play and then an indeterminate amount of time asleep. They are instead broken up into ninety-minute cycles to build harmony between activity and recovery.

Your fixed wake time provides the anchor around which all of your day is structured. In the diagram opposite, the wake time is 6:30 a.m., but yours could be whenever you choose. Just count back in ninety-minute cycles for your sleep times. In this instance, an ideal five-cycle routine involves being asleep by 11 p.m. It can move later to 12:30 a.m. if your life demands it at the time, or later still to 2 a.m. No need to worry about *enough* sleep, because it's just one night out of seven, and your ninety-minute pre- and post-sleep routines, as well as your controlled recovery room and tailored sleep kit, are going to ensure you get the right *quality* of recovery. You are going to

The R90 Day for a 6:30 Wake Time

take a break every ninety minutes, even if it's just to walk out-side tech-free, go to the bathroom, or get a drink. You also have two windows of opportunity that can help, either a ninety- or thirty-minute Controlled Recovery Period in the midday slot or a thirty-minute CRP in the early evening slot. You're in control of this.

You then take this daily outlook into a longer period of time. You can look at it as part of a weekly schedule, in which you know that, if you are the type who needs five cycles per night, an ideal week is thirty-five cycles. For you, twenty-eight is OK, but anything less and you might be pushing it—it's a po-tential red flag. You could keep a very simple diary, recording only measurable data.

JESS'S SLEEP PLANNER

	Activity	Cycles
Monday	*Working late on presentation*	CRP: Nocturnal: 4
Tuesday	*Dinner after work with the girls*	CRP: 1 (30 min midday) Nocturnal: 4
Wednesday	*Running club*	CRP: 1 (30 min midday) Nocturnal: 4
Thursday	*Carl's going-away drinks*	CRP: 1 (30 min early evening) Nocturnal: 3
Friday		CRP: Nocturnal: 5
Saturday	*House party!*	CRP: 1 (30 min early evening) Nocturnal: 2
Sunday	*Movies @ 9*	CRP: 1 (90 min midday) Nocturnal: 4

On this particular week, Jess, who has a Monday-to-Friday job in an office and whose ideal routine is thirty-five cycles, manages to get thirty-one. She will certainly be feeling the effects of only two cycles on Saturday night before getting up at her constant wake time of 6:30 on Sunday, but she copes: she gets up, has her breakfast, and goes for a walk before returning home to slump on the sofa and catch up on her favorite guilty pleasures on television. In the midday window, with no work to interfere, she closes her recovery room's blackout blinds, sets the alarm, and has a ninety-minute CRP in her sleep kit.

She's achieving her ideal amount of five cycles four times in this week, and she makes sure to follow two consecutive nights of fewer cycles with her ideal. There is nothing in Jess's diary that would worry me hugely if I were working with her, but if she should start feeling below par or a bit tired after her week, with the help of her sleep schedule she can start to understand why. She can look to change things the following week and achieve more cycles in better harmony by looking at what is negotiable time. Her running club is her main form of exercise, so that's non-negotiable, and who wants to leave a party early if they're having a great time? But perhaps she could look to cancel the movie date on a Sunday night or go to an earlier screening next time, and find a way to use CRPs more regularly.

Knowing that you can do something about your sleep in this way is empowering. You have measurable data at your disposal to make adjustments that will benefit the way you feel and perform. Start looking at your week ahead, allocating your recovery periods, estimating the number of cycles you will get. Is that enough? Can you get an extra CRP in here or there? Plans change, impromptu social opportunities and work demands crop up, but you can be flexible. You can move your sleep time, get another CRP in, use those ninety-minute recovery breaks, get daylight or daylight lamps on you to stay ahead of the game. You're doing your preparation early, putting yourself in control.

Those who don't have the head start that the R90 offers are still sleepwalking through a random approach to their recovery. They feel tired, they know they're not getting enough sleep, but what are they going to do about it? They don't have any real measure of how much they're getting, and they don't have the approach as well as the sleep kit and recovery room you've built up to ensure that they are getting the right quality. They might set the alarm for a little later than usual; they might go to bed earlier than usual; they might nod off on the train home from work or at their desk. But there is no strategy behind this. They don't have the tools to improve their day-to-day life, so they stumble through, taking actions that seem intuitively to be correct (need more rest = sleep longer) but that are in fact counterproductive. Changing your wake time and going to bed too early aren't helping, so stop doing those things. If you need more rest, sleep *smarter*.

Eat a Healthy Diet, Exercise Regularly— and Recover Well

In terms of the information we are fed from governments, doctors, and health organizations around the world, a healthy lifestyle consists of a good, balanced diet and plenty of physical activity. The American Heart Association produced a set of diet and lifestyle guidelines to reduce cardiovascular risk in 2013, which includes detailed advice on food and exercise amounts and warns of the perils of alcohol and smoking.[1] The World Health Organization's 2004 Global Strategy on Diet, Physical Activity and Health is an approach to tackling non-communicable diseases such as cancer, obesity, and type 2 diabetes.

You can find excellent advice and the very best of intentions in these publications, along with the countless others produced around the world, with just one caveat: where's the sleep section? The link between sleep and cardiovascular problems has already been made,[2] and there is an increasing amount of research demonstrating the effect sleep has on cancer, obesity, and diabetes. So, wouldn't it make sense to include information on sleep?

Recovery should be the third part of our approach to healthy living. The benefits I see on a daily basis in those practicing the R90 program can be just as powerful as the other two, but they are benefits that can only really be enjoyed in harmony with a good diet and exercise. If you eat poorly and don't exercise, it's going to cause problems. Getting these things right will improve the quality of your sleep and, as part of a three-pronged approach, improve the quality of your life immeasurably.

Obviously, the athletes I work with are super-fit and eat a controlled diet tailored to their needs. And it's often the very best of these athletes, who have the attitude that being the best entails, who show the greatest commitment to recovery.

When I started at Manchester United in the 1990s, a young Ryan Giggs was one of the first players to really show an interest in what I was doing. This wasn't the yoga-practicing Ryan that the soccer world is familiar with today, but it was a good demonstration of the kind of intellectual curiosity and openness to new ideas that would lead to this and to his playing at the top level long after the average player hung up their cleats.

You see this in all the best athletes. I saw it in Gareth Bale and Cristiano Ronaldo at Real Madrid, and in the likes of Bradley Wiggins and Chris Hoy. I see it in youth-level prospects you've yet to hear of. If you take your diet and exercise seriously and you've read this far, you share some of this attitude too.

Diet

If the R90 program is a revolutionary approach to your sleep, adopting a suitable diet in coordination with your rest is anything but. Chances are you already have thought about your diet. Eating as broad a range of fresh foods as possible; avoiding food grown, treated, or processed with chemicals; being aware of any food allergies; and, in particular, controlling your salt, sugar (your body will crave this if you're not sleeping well), calorie, and caffeine intake—all these are well-documented, sensible habits.

Hydrating with the correct amount of water is important. Everyone is different, and your activity throughout the day will affect this, so don't blindly down eight glasses per day because of the latest recommendations that make the news. Athletes don't do this. They know that there is water present in food, particularly in vegetable-rich diets, so they make adjustments for this. It's not rocket science: listen to your body and drink regularly throughout the day when you're thirsty, especially after exercise. The amount of liquid we consume becomes particularly important as we approach our designated sleep time. If you take on too much, it could wake you up during the night.

Tryptophan is an essential amino acid found in protein-rich foods such as chicken, turkey, cheese, fish, milk, and nuts, as well as in some other foods such as bananas. Our bodies use it as a component in serotonin production, and consequently melatonin, so get plenty of it in your diet.

One of the latest biohacks being used in sports is Montmorency tart cherries. These are available fresh, frozen, dried, or as a juice, and they are worth tracking down even when fresh cherries aren't in season (just make sure you're getting the right variety!). Glyn Howatson of Northumbria University has led numerous studies demonstrating their benefits on recovery after strenuous exercise, with one such piece of research proving that the cherries produce an increase in melatonin, which is "beneficial in improving sleep duration and quality in healthy men and women and might be of benefit in managing disturbed sleep."[3]

You should aim to eat your final meal of the day two cycles (three hours) before your targeted sleep time, and any last light snack ninety minutes before, at the beginning of your pre-sleep routine. Eating "too late" simply means eating too close to your targeted sleep time. If you're eating at 9 p.m. and your wake time is 6:30 a.m., move a cycle later from 11 p.m. and target 12:30 a.m. as your sleep time. There's no such thing as too late when it's part of a controlled approach, although eating late as a habit may interfere with your circadian rhythms.

Our bodies love patterns and harmonies. Your circadian rhythms can also be influenced by eating times, so getting some harmony with this, starting with breakfast, will help, along with your regular wake time. Remember, a good diet isn't necessarily about eating foods that will help you sleep well (though it's certainly about avoiding those that will prevent you from sleeping well); rather, it involves combining that with good sleeping habits and exercise so you feel at your best every day.

Exercise

While sleep is taken for granted by many people in our day-to-day lives, it's easier for me to take exercise for granted when I work with sports people. Exercise is their job, after all.

We've already talked about the importance of some exercise as part of your post- and pre-sleep routines, to get your body started for the day and to prepare you better for your sleep time.

But on top of this, a regular exercise regimen offers considerable benefits to your sleep. An Oregon State University study put the improvement in sleep quality from 150 minutes of moderate to vigorous exercise per week at 65 percent.[4] It's unlikely you need such a study to inform you of these benefits. When we've exercised during the day, we tend to get into our sleep kit with our bodies nicely tired and just drift away.

A real gym culture has developed in Western society, certainly over the last twenty or thirty years. In the United States alone, the number of memberships at gyms and health clubs has increased from 32.8 million to 55 million since 2000.[5] Many of the sports and fitness conferences I speak at are packed full of people bouncing on trampolines, blasting the exercise bikes, and looking hungrily for the latest equipment or exercise technique in their quest for physical perfection. This embracing of the gym is fantastic, but it's not for everyone—nor does it have to be.

Some people just can't get along with the gym. They'd rather do yoga or Pilates, or be outside running, cycling, swimming, or participating in all manner of exotic and ever-changing exercise classes (including yoga and Pilates, when the weather allows). These are all excellent options too, particularly being outdoors, as it can give us a welcome dose of daylight (depending on the time we do it).

There are those whose motivation to get and stay fit is to play a sport. Professional sports people fall into this camp, of course. They might love playing football for a living, but they don't always love the training and fitness work that goes into it, and it's not uncommon to see a retired football player or a boxer who's between bouts ease up on their routine and put on a few pounds. For others, it's playing golf that keeps them fit, or gardening, or going for a good walk with the dog every day. It could even be commuting to work on a bicycle rather than the bus.

The point is that there should be something for everyone when it comes to being active. And another great benefit is that we can use the time we spend exercising to give ourselves a mind break, just tuning out as we clock up the miles on the treadmill or the laps in the pool. If we're able to give ourselves a tech break too, then all the better. This doesn't have to mean leaving your smartphone behind if you use it to measure your running progress or your King of the Mountain status on Strava. It could just mean setting it to "do not disturb" so that you're not engaging with the outside world.

It's best not to do any strenuous exercise close to sleep, as you will need time to come down from the attendant adrenaline surge and raised heart rate. And be aware of your circadian rhythms if you want to start setting personal bests: most world records in athletics, including cycling, are broken in the afternoon and evening.

Recovering from your exercise is vital. Factor in recovery periods, hydrate and fuel up when required, and use supplements and biohacks like Montmorency tart cherries to help. The comfort of your sleep kit becomes extra important if you do intense exercise and you have aching joints and limbs. The surface needs to give sufficiently so that it doesn't exacerbate any pain that might stop you from getting to sleep—or leave you feeling even worse in the morning. Getting your ideal amount of cycles that night and using CRPs are sound ideas too.

I work with Michael Torres, a fitness expert whose company, SHIFT Performance, is at the forefront of the human performance industry. As he says, "Personally, my view of recovery has broadened over years from the integration of massage therapy to monitoring sleep, performance, and stress, and more recently diving into sleep as a recovery system.

"Recovery is the common denominator that affects all things. We have explored recovery as much more of a training program element, not something outside of the training cycle. This is the future."

Electric Dreams

You wake up just before your alarm goes off. You get up, turn it off, open the blackout blinds. It's a glorious day. You go to the bathroom, empty your bladder, then go to the kitchen to make some breakfast. You eat outside, feeling yourself wake gradually in the sunshine as you listen to the birds sing. You shower and ready yourself for work. You feel alert and good, rested and ready for the day ahead—you can't wait to get started. You pick up your smartphone and check your sleep app to see how you performed last night. It says you had a terrible night's sleep. Too much light sleep, not enough of the deep stuff. In your app's eyes, the day is practically a write-off.

Wearable fitness trackers, which record data such as steps taken, calories burned, and type of activity, are a huge, growing market, predicted to be worth over $5 billion by 2019 (up from $2 billion in 2014).[6] Products such as Fitbit and Jawbone have become household names to many, and with companies like Apple joining the market with their Apple Watch, we've never been more motivated in our hunt for data to support our fitness and health. These trackers, along with various apps available on smartphones, also claim to measure sleep.

Utilizing performance data is a vital part of modern sports, and wearable trackers such as those produced by Whoop, a company that tailors them for athletes, play a part in this, particularly in flagging the potential for injury when an athlete is pushing it too much. The performers sometimes grumble about using them, as they feel they aren't in complete control of the data, but they generally accept it as part of the job.

When it comes to tracking sleep data, however, things become a bit muddier. Professional athletes quite rightly think of the time they spend away from their work as their own, and they can be resistant to having their sleep monitored. If an elite performer has their boyfriend or girlfriend over for an early night but a late sleep time, they consider it their own business, not the team's or coach's. This is their private time, and athletes can be apt to think that their employer is trying to control them if it's not handled correctly. You might have little sympathy for this situation, given the amount some top sports people earn, but how would you feel if your employer asked you to wear a wristband so they could monitor what you get up to every night?

This might be more pertinent to you than you imagine, as fitness tracker information has been used in legal proceedings.

When I'm working with a team, we will ask athletes to wear the devices for a specific period, and then *we*, not the athlete, collect the data. We don't want any data-based doubt creeping into their heads first thing in the morning, just as you don't want to allow any data to compromise how you feel when you wake up. We then use the data to advise the athlete in practical terms how they can improve their recovery routines. Just as we do with the fitness data, we use the wearables to spot red flags in sleeping habits. If there are indications of health risks, such as a player is overdoing it or there's an undiagnosed condition like sleep apnea, we can make an intervention. I'm not there to play Big Brother to them.

The problem with many of the wearables and apps available for use at home is that they provide their information through an accelerometer, which basically captures motion. Moving a lot indicates light sleep; no movement, deep sleep. While the wearable device can at least guarantee that all the movement is yours, the apps, with your phone placed strategically by the side of the bed, aren't so accurate. If the person you're sharing a bed with gets in the way, it records that. If your dog jumps on the bed—please don't tell me you share your recovery room with a pet—it records that too.

Where apps have the potential to be of more use is as an education tool. I have helped Southampton Football Club overhaul their app for players and staff, introducing new sections in their questionnaires to better evaluate the recovery habits of players and offer them tailored, practical advice to improve their regimens.

The role of wearable and sleep-monitoring technology is helpful in some ways, because at least it is getting people talking about the subject of sleep. It's opening up some awareness and providing some limited knowledge on sleep stages and the importance of deep sleep. The reality, however, is that once the novelty wears off, the information the devices provide rarely has an impact on people's lives, and so they stop using it. If you wake up feeling refreshed and ready for the day ahead but your app says you slept poorly, who are you going to believe?

Only a polysomnogram—in which things like brain wave activity, eye movement, and muscle movement are monitored—can accurately record the stages within sleeping cycles. But the devices are certainly getting more sophisticated, measuring heart rate and temperature as well as motion. A device called the Zeo, a headband measuring electrical signals in your brain, promised to measure sleep stages more accurately, but it's no longer commercially available.

The simple fact is that while this technology can provide some kind of guide as to how you *might* be sleeping, you would be far better off investing your money in some of the things we have talked about so far in this book if you actually want to do something definite about improving the quality of your sleep. Upgrading your sleep kit, a dawn simulator, blackout blinds, and red bulbs for your lamps are all better uses of your money. And downloading a meditation app instead of one that promises to measure your sleep is certainly a better use of your time too.

The Three-Pronged Attack

The image I always return to when looking at sleep in conjunction with diet and exercise is one of an Italian family sitting around a table outside in an olive grove. The sun is shining. There are fresh fruit and vegetables on the table, a carafe of red wine, and some cheese and freshly made bread. The family includes several generations, from the children to the old man at the head of the table, still spry and active in his weather-beaten skin, pouring the wine and laughing and joking with his grandchildren. Do you think he sleeps well as he dozes in the shade later on?

There's no sign of a gym, with its pounding music and strobe lighting. It's just a family doing the simple things right in their own environment. But it doesn't matter if you live in a house in the suburbs or an apartment on the twentieth floor of a high-rise in a city, if you work 9–5 in an office or on a construction site—*anyone* can make their own version of this image. You can find the exercise and activity regimen that works for you. You can eat a balanced, healthy diet. There's no need to become obsessive about it—there's still room for a piece of cake and a glass of wine when you want one—and you can integrate the R90 program into your life, so you recover properly and make the most out of every day. Because if you get this right, you're going to feel terrific.

NINE

Sleeping with the Enemy

Sleep Problems

Spring is in the air. The clocks are going to move forward soon. Rebecca recently moved her wake time earlier, to 5 a.m., as part of her tailored R90 program.[1] What might be even more surprising to read is that she's about to start a three-cycle routine.

When she first got in touch, Rebecca was struggling. She has a high-pressure job in banking, but she lived within walking distance of her office, so she was able to go to the gym first thing in the morning and have a positive start to her day before work. Then her office moved across town, her commute increased several times over, and she stopped going to the gym. She didn't have the time.

Rebecca had always been a sensitive sleeper, waking up a lot during the night and having trouble with her breathing in the form of asthma and allergies. She'd been like that for as long as she could remember. Once that great, stress-busting, energizing start to the day at the gym was out of the picture, she started to feel worse in her day-to-day life: fatigued and irritable, with low mood and motivation, relying increasingly on caffeine and sugary snacks to push on through. She was then struggling to get to sleep and waking increasingly often during the night, which fueled her fatigue, irritability, low mood, and lack of motivation in a vicious circle.

She had spent hours online researching her symptoms, had been to the doctor, and had even seen a specialist, but they were unable to diagnose anything specific or provide anything practical for use in her everyday life. She was trying herbal teas, relaxing baths, and over-the-counter sleep aids—and then sleeping pills. But none of it was having any impact. Finally her partner started sleeping on the sofa bed until she figured it out.

When she contacted me I first asked her to fill in the R90 sleep profile questionnaire I use, designed to provide a complete picture of the subject's everyday life—what they are doing, when, and why. It isn't full of multiple-choice questions asking, "How long do you wake up for during the night: fifteen, thirty, forty-five, sixty minutes or longer?" because, frankly, who on earth can answer questions like that accurately? Instead, I ask questions with a definite answer, often just a yes or no. *Are you aware of circadian rhythms? Do you know your chronotype? Do you wake up during the night* at all? She also sent in photographs of her mattress and her sleeping environment. (Even for photographs, most people, just like football player Rod and his wife in Chapter 7, make sure their bedroom is tidy and looking its best.)

I could see immediately that she had a large bedroom but just a standard full-size bed. "Have you thought about getting a bigger bed?" I asked. She was sleeping on a pocketed-coil mattress with natural filler. "What about getting something hypoallergenic for your asthma?" I suggested. She quickly became familiar with cycles and rhythms, and soon she started to feel a bit more positive about things. And then we used this knowledge to help her start making some gains in her life.

She packed away the sleeping aids. She was used to getting up at 6 a.m. for work and going to bed at 10 p.m. on an "ideal" night, but, as she's an AMer and with summer not too far away and the lighter mornings that would bring, we gave her a constant wake time of 5. The sun will be up around then, so it won't hurt an AM chronotype to do something like that. Then we counted back in ninety-minute cycles to give her potential sleep times of 3:30 a.m., 2 a.m., 12:30 a.m., and 11 p.m. It's no good using 9:30 p.m., because with the clocks changing the sun will have barely gone down then, and the circadian urge and sleep pressure peak later in the evening. If she needs five cycles, we can use CRPs or her wake time will have to move to 6:30 a.m.

She can go to the gym again, and start her day on the right foot. She's starting to feel better at work, and more empowered as she adopts her own R90 program, shopping around to build her sleep kit and manage her environment better. She uses her targeted sleep time of 11 p.m., by which time she's tired and falls asleep OK, but she is still waking up during the night. I ask her if she's ever considered the idea that around eight hours might not actually be right for her. Instead of lying there tossing and turning, maybe she's the round-the-world-sailor or Yahoo CEO Marissa Mayer type, who needs less sleep than most.

So, having adjusted well to her new wake time, she looks surprised when I suggest she start going to bed at 12:30 a.m. *Only three cycles?*

Restriction

When people I work with tell me they wake up and get up during the night, that's an immediate red flag. It doesn't matter whether it's for five minutes or an hour—I don't want you waking up at all during the night.

Much of what we addressed in the Key Sleep Recovery Indicators showed how to push aside as many of the obstacles as possible to transitioning smoothly through our cycles at night. We've talked throughout this book about the potential for stress and worry about sleep to keep us awake, and how looking at it in a broader time frame and knowing you can do something about it in your waking hours to adjust can help.

Using ninety-minute cycles in the R90 program provides us with our very own DIY polysomnogram that we can use when we are having trouble with our sleep. If we wake at the start or end of a cycle during the night (looking at a clock should confirm this), then we know that if we don't go back to sleep reasonably swiftly afterward, we can get up, do some pre-sleep activities, and try to catch the next cycle. We can look at what might have woken us up. If it's going to the bathroom, did we drink too much liquid the day before? Did we consume more caffeine the day before? Is anything stressful going on? There's nothing random in our approach—just some very simple self-diagnoses.

If we wake up midcycle, we can get up and aim to sleep for the start of the next cycle. We're in control. If we wake up too early, in the last cycle before our scheduled wake time, we can relax in bed until our fixed wake time and then kick-start our day. If this waking can be attributed to a specific incident, we can target a sleep time a cycle later so that we can aim to sleep through rather than experience disrupted sleep. If sleeping problems still persist, we can turn to the process of sleep restriction.

Sleep restriction sounds counterintuitive at first. If you're having trouble sleeping, feeling exhausted in the day, how is restricting it going to help? But in fact it works on a very simple premise: if you aren't getting enough sleep but you're wasting your time in bed trying, let's cut down on the time you're wasting. Let's make that time in bed *efficient* time.

So because Rebecca, whose targeted sleep time was 11 p.m. and wake time was 5 a.m., was still waking in the night and struggling to get back to sleep, we'd move her to a 12:30 sleep time and see how she fared.

The biggest barrier is often psychological. After years of blindly accepting that we should spend eight hours in bed a night, it's difficult to retrain the mind to accept that four and a half hours will be enough. But what is going to be more beneficial: three smoothly transitioning cycles with at least a good portion of the relevant stages of sleep (remember, your mind will prioritize REM if you haven't been getting enough), or a similar amount of sleep broken up and spread thinly across eight hours in which light sleep dominates?

Rebecca might find it difficult to stay up until after midnight; she will naturally get tired and want to go to sleep sooner. But it is vital for her to resist this. Doing some gentle exercise such as going for a walk and getting some fresh air will help perk her up so that she can make it through. Keeping active until later is key, so she shouldn't spend all night on the sofa in front of the television. The wake time, as ever, is a constant.

She might well feel fatigued during the day. It is important that she has the maximum amount of pre- and post-sleep routine she can manage (ninety minutes, ideally), uses her breaks every ninety minutes and CRPs when needed, and gets as much daylight on her as possible during these periods to give her a boost and reset her body clock.

With the R90 program, we look at our sleep in schedules of seven days, not one night, so if after seven days she's still experiencing problems, we could go down another cycle, to a sleep time of 2 a.m. This might sound incredible, but it's important to realize that it isn't designed to be a long-term measure. It's effectively about resetting your sleep pattern, getting you down to rock bottom in terms of the amount of time you are able to sleep efficiently, so that we can then start building it back up.

If a sleep pattern of 2 until 5 a.m. finally works for Rebecca, she will start to see some other benefits. As she's being dumped straight into sleep—at the time when our circadian urge is at its strongest—and remaining in it solidly for two cycles, she might soon find she no longer needs earplugs, as she isn't in that light-sleep stage, from which we can easily be roused, for as long. She might even discover that she's in the short-sleeping group of people—who make up 1 percent of the population.

What it does give her is a base from which she knows she can confidently achieve three hours of uninterrupted sleep. If you are the type who sleeps soundly through your five cycles per night, this will mean little to you, but for some people, after years of broken sleep, it is an incredibly powerful starting point. We would keep her on it for seven days, monitor it, and then come back to a 12:30 sleep time. Or if during the course of adopting this regimen she has started going to the gym after work to keep her going for longer into the evening, we could move her constant wake time to 6:30. This is a positive action. She has changed her routine to find time in the evening for the gym because she now goes to bed later, and she is sleeping through without constant interruptions.

She would settle into this routine for seven days and, assuming it worked, then we would look to move it back again, so that she is on a four-cycle routine. Eleven p.m. until 5 a.m. (or 12:30–6:30)—six hours per night—suddenly doesn't sound so bad. She didn't know how much sleep she was getting before, how much she really needed, but now she's starting to see.

Sleep restriction isn't an overnight process, so it's disappointing when I have clients who come to me after they have been on a restriction regimen in which, if they slept through one night without waking, they would move their targeted sleep time fifteen minutes earlier; if they didn't, they moved it fifteen minutes later. In my experience, this approach is too erratic and puts on too much pressure, leaving its participants feeling like they're indulging in a mean-spirited video game: get tonight right if you want to proceed to the next level, but if you fail, go back to the previous one.

Alleviating this idea that one night is everything is so important when dealing with disturbed sleep. It's why I look at cycles per week and preach a 24/7 recovery schedule, because it's not fair to have so much riding on tonight. When sleep is restricted without these parameters and it is done consistently over a larger sample size of seven nights rather than just one, then we can look to build confidence in the knowledge that it's only one night out of several. It's part of a gradual routine change, not a challenge with penalties and rewards.

Insomnia

Insomnia is the daddy of sleeping problems. It is the first thing most of us think of when we talk of such matters, and it seems an unlikely word to appear for the first time so late in a book on sleep.

In fact, insomnia is a word that describes a whole host of sleeping conditions in which the sufferer experiences trouble either falling asleep or staying asleep, and that impairs the ability to function in the waking hours. According to Chris Idzikowski, one of my valued industry mentors and a former adviser to the UK Sleep Council, "insomnia is caused by hyperarousal, a state in which a person's brain is simply too excited to sleep."[2]

For some people, this might mean that a period of stress, such as a bereavement or difficult times at work, causes them to struggle with short-term insomnia. For others, there is the long-term problem of chronic insomnia, a serious condition that might have no obvious cause or might be a marker for other problems such as anxiety disorders and depression.

A colleague of mine suffers from chronic insomnia. He's lucky to get an hour of sleep per night. When he suffered from it originally, his body would simply crash during the day: he'd collapse straight into sleep anywhere, even in the street. Quite literally a waking nightmare for him. But he has adjusted now, and while his amount of sleep has not improved, his ability to deal with it has. Our bodies and minds adapt. He now uses the time to get two days' work done in a day, particularly handy when working with people in different time zones. When we used a sleep-tracking device called Zeo on him, which allowed us to monitor his brain-wave patterns, we picked up the kind of activity associated with a sleeping stage . . . while he was busy sending emails. To me, it suggests the possibility that his brain could be resting in some form while he is awake during the night, though his diagnosis is much simpler: the machine doesn't work.

This kind of chronic insomnia, or the kind that suggests a mental health condition, has a very simple recommendation from me: see a doctor. It warrants a clinical diagnosis and medical attention. However, for those suffering from other types of insomnia—which I prefer simply to think of in terms of trouble getting to sleep or waking up during the night—the R90 program is an effective tool. Pre- and post-sleep routines, the constant wake time, harmony with the body clock, a properly prepared sleep environment, regular breaks, and exercise can all help, and the process of sleep restriction is a method used not only by me but also by health-care providers around the world. If this is unsuccessful, then see a doctor, but, given the workload of many medical professionals, it could be that they'll simply write you a prescription for something to help you sleep. And that might be where your troubles begin.

The Drugs Don't Work

With all the pressures, adrenaline, and use—and overuse—of caffeine in sports, it is little surprise that there is a culture of using sleeping pills in many of the teams I work with. What goes up must come down, after all.

The global sleep aids market was valued at $58.1 billion in 2014 and is expected to be worth more like $80.8 billion in 2020.[3] A recent report put the number of American adults taking prescription sleep aids at around 9 million, with their use tripling between 1998 and 2006 in those between eighteen and twenty-four years of age.[4]

The dangers of misusing these drugs are significant, with emergency room visits involving zolpidem (a hypnotic—a drug that acts on the nervous system to induce sleep—that is the active ingredient in sleeping pills such as America's most popular option, Ambien) almost doubling between 2005 and 2010. Sleeping pills can be habit-forming, can induce memory loss and sleepwalking—with some extreme stories of people waking up having been sleepdriving, with catastrophic results—and they can stay in the body longer than you might expect, affecting balance, alertness, and reaction times the day after.[5] They are certainly not a performance enhancer in this sense.

A study in 2012 drawing a link between sleeping pills and mortality and cancer reported "substantially elevated hazards of dying compared to those prescribed no hypnotics," even in those who took relatively few pills.[6] So, are the risks worth it? A study of Z drugs—the group of hypnotics to which zolpidem belongs—reported an improvement of only twenty-two minutes in the length of time it took the subjects to get to sleep compared to a placebo.[7]

Drugs are not the answer to persistent sleep problems. They are effective in helping short-term cases of insomnia, such as those caused by grief or similarly traumatic events, and the National Health Service in the United Kingdom recommends that they should be used in treatments only up to four weeks. However, Kevin Morgan of Loughborough University's Sleep Research Centre says, "Most clinical insomnias are chronic, so most of these drugs are prescribed for longer than they should."

But why bother with a prescription? Many sleeping pills are readily available online without need of one, which means people who are effectively self-diagnosing sleeping conditions are using powerful and potentially habit-forming drugs unsupervised by a medical professional. The UK Sleep Council's *Great British Bedtime Report* in 2013 showed that while one in ten people had consulted their doctor about sleeping problems, three times that number had taken medication to help them sleep.

Here's some very straightforward advice about sleep aids: stop using them. Right now. Unless you have a diagnosed sleeping or mental health condition and they are a necessary part of your treatment, they are doing you no good. They have the power to be psychologically addictive. They can form part of an unwanted pre-sleep routine in which the user has become so familiar with the habit of taking them before they go to sleep that they become convinced they can't sleep without them. If they try to sleep without this crutch they've come to rely on, anxiety will strike and they'll be kept awake by unhelpful thoughts, fueling the idea that they're reliant upon them.

One of the first jobs I will be tasked with when I start working with a sports team is to get the athletes off sleeping pills. The team doctor might already have tried, with their words falling on deaf ears. But the doctor knows those medications are taking a toll. "I need them. I can't sleep the night before or after a game," might come the player's reply.

"Then don't bother," I say. "If you can't sleep, find other ways to recover. Meditate. Watch a highlights reel of your best moments in your sport. Use the time for other things." Watching themselves perform at their best can help settle some of the anxiety that might be preventing them from sleeping, giving them confidence for the upcoming performance. When British Olympian Steve Redgrave couldn't sleep before he competed, it didn't worry him. He'd still go out, row like a man possessed, finish first, and then recover afterward.

If you're struggling to sleep, why not do something similar to give you a bit of confidence and feel better about things? You might not have a highlights reel to watch, but surely you can play something back in your head that you could draw confidence from. It's got to be better than thinking about not sleeping. Get up, do something akin to another pre-sleep routine—meditate, listen to something relaxing on your headphones—and then see if you can aim to sleep at the start of another cycle (so if you're struggling to sleep around 1 a.m. and your wake time is 6:30, either 2 or 3:30 would be the next natural entry point for sleep). Take control of your situation and take proactive steps to address it.

Rebecca, mentioned at the start of the chapter, used over-the-counter sleep aids to try to deal with her problem.[8] These drugs accounted for $428 million in sales in the United States in 2016.[9] Over-the-counter sleep aids, which often use antihistamines as the active ingredient, have limited use in isolation. The placebo effect—*I'm taking a pill; therefore I can reduce my anxiety about sleep*—can be powerful, as has been found in trials with more potent prescription aids, and many people are apt to forget the steps they take around using a sleeping aid for the first night or two. Having recognized that they need something to help them sleep, they will probably cut down on the unhelpful elements of their lifestyle that night, such as drinking alcohol and being out late, and maybe reduce their caffeine intake during the day. They might continue this for a night or two and get some better sleep, but once they revert back to their usual lifestyle, the product will show itself to be nothing other than a short-term balm. A short-term balm can still be useful when used as part of a coordinated approach, of course, and these nonprescription sleep aids are certainly not likely to cause the problems more potent prescription medications can. But if you want to see more regular results, the R90 program is a far more reliable long-term sleeping aid than any pill.

Jet Lag

The first leg of my flight to Australia took off from Birmingham airport at 9 p.m. I had a meal, watched a movie, then pushed the button to turn my seat into a bed (business class was one of the perks of being flown out there for work) and slept for the rest of the flight, touching down in Dubai at 7 a.m. local time. I stayed up for the day, met up with my friend Andy Oldknow, who lives in Dubai, had an evening meal with him, and then returned to the airport for the 2 a.m. flight on to Sydney.[10] Thirteen hours later, having slept on the plane for a few hours, I landed in the evening. I arrived at my hotel, had something to eat, relaxed for a while, and went to bed with the alarm set for the morning, as I had to be at a television studio at 11 a.m. I had been following a fairly normal routine, despite the jumps in time zones, and I slept soundly that night.

In the morning I felt fine—not 100 percent, of course, but then I'd spent a long time traveling and there's always going to be a bit of residual fatigue (long-distance travel in itself is tiring, especially spending several hours in a cramped space, and this can sometimes be difficult to differentiate from jet-lag symptoms). I arrived at the TV studio in plenty of time, and as I prepared for my piece, everything was OK . . . until I just completely shut down with the cameras on me. By the third take, I couldn't even speak. Everything went fuzzy and felt out of kilter with what I would consider a normal version of reality. I could not push past it, so, having flown around the world to do this very piece of TV work, I had to go back to my hotel. How on earth did that happen?

When we travel a long distance rapidly east or west across time zones, our circadian rhythms struggle with being out of sync with the light-dark cycle of the new environment, and we experience jet lag. Evolution has yet to catch up with the invention of the jet engine.

Disrupted sleep patterns—trouble falling asleep and staying asleep—and enhanced daytime levels of fatigue are the usual signs of jet lag. We're alert and then tired at all the wrong times while our body clock adapts. Matters are further complicated by the fact that even once the master body clock in the brain has adjusted to the light-dark schedule, the individual clocks in our cells and organs controlled by our master clock all need to recalibrate.

The farther you travel and the greater the time difference, the more acute the impact is likely to be. As a very rough rule of thumb, it is estimated that it takes a day for every hour's difference to adjust, but it affects different people to different degrees. We could fly a team of thirty soccer players out to the Far East for a preseason promotional tournament, with all of them following the same regimen and using the same interventions, and half the players might be fine to play the day after landing, while the others would be wiped out. The truth is that we can put steps in place to attempt to prepare us better for it, but it's no guarantee we'll be spared. On my flight to Australia, I enjoyed the luxury of business class, so I was better able to sleep at the right times than I would have been in a cramped economy-class section, and I was able to bring all my experience in sleep to bear—but I still crashed.

Those of us who have been on vacations that involve long-haul travel are likely to have experienced jet lag, and it can disrupt the start of a trip as well as our reintegration into our day-to-day life when we return home. When we're on vacation, the symptoms might be unwelcome, but if we're relaxing on a beach, they aren't going to cause too many problems. For people flying out on business or returning back to work after a vacation, however, the impact can be more damaging. The symptoms need to be managed.

The most effective treatment for jet lag is, of course, time. Athletes at the Rio Olympics didn't fly in the day before their event, nor did any of the soccer teams arrive the day before their first match at the World Cup in Brazil in 2014. They arrived in plenty of time for their circadian rhythms to adjust to the local light-dark schedule. If you are able to fly out in advance of a meeting or have a day or two off from work after you return from your vacation, it would help, but the modern demands of business and the high value we place on our annual time off usually mean this isn't an option.

In the NBA and NFL, teams have to travel across time zones within the United States for games, so jet lag can become a factor in games where East Coast teams play West Coast rivals. Given the more regular demands of domestic league games compared to every-four-year events like the Olympics and the World Cup, time isn't on their side, so they have to use other measures to combat it.

Some airlines have their own jet-lag apps or online advisers, which can be of help, but as ever, light is our most potent weapon. We can use light before, during, and after our flight to reset our body clocks and help offset the effects of jet lag. Adopting a very simple pre-adaptation routine before you fly allows you to get a head start. If you are flying from New York to London, which means five time zones east (five hours ahead), you would need to move your body clock *earlier* to start matching the time zone at your destination. Traveling east is generally considered to be more difficult than traveling west, so some preparation is especially recommended when heading this way. You could start to move your wake time and sleep time earlier each day for a couple of days before, using light—either natural or from a daylight lamp—earlier in the morning and avoiding light and targeting an earlier sleep time that night.

The same logic would follow the trip in reverse (London to New York), with the journey west meaning you would use light for an hour in the evening to keep you awake longer, so you could target a later sleep time and a later wake time the following morning before your flight to move toward the time of your destination.

On the plane, use light if the daylight hours of your destination require it. While packing a daylight lamp in your carry-on isn't an option, you could use a product such as Human Charger, a jet-lag aid that will give you light through your ear canals and won't look any more conspicuous than if you were just listening to some music.

Adapting to the new destination is as much about avoiding light as it is about exposing yourself to it. Avoid light on the plane in accordance with the daylight hours of your destination—keep your window blind shut when it's daylight outside if you're able to, or use an eye mask or even sunglasses, which might draw some funny looks from fellow passengers (unless you're in first class, in which case they'll just assume you're famous).

Once you're at your destination, you can continue to phase in your adjustment by moving your clock earlier or later gradually each day, using sunglasses, blackout, and staying indoors to avoid light, and getting daylight on you at the right times, though by this time you might just find it practical to adopt the daylight hours of your destination. If you have trouble sleeping at your destination and you get up during the night, avoid any activities that involve bright light; similarly, during the day make sure you get plenty of daylight on you and avoid sleeping the whole day in blackout. If you've done some preparation work, the effects of jet lag shouldn't be as severe or last as long.

Light is of particular benefit if we're flying straight in for a meeting or event and we're not able to phase in the changes to our body clocks. Its ability to boost mood and alertness means we can use daylight devices, as well as controlled doses of caffeine, to give us a fix to get us through the main event; if we crash after it's all over, it isn't so important. Light is a far more effective natural weapon against jet lag than overstimulating on caffeine and using sleeping pills. Looking after yourself by staying hydrated and avoiding alcohol, which won't really help you sleep, on the plane are important too.

The International Air Transport Association published results in 2015 showing that global passenger traffic had increased by 6.5 percent over the year before, so our demand for it certainly isn't going away. If you're a regular flyer, taking some steps to find what works for you means that jet lag doesn't have to inhibit your performance. Even if you're an infrequent flyer, being sharp back at work the day after you land is going to be possible only if you look after yourself when you travel.

If some of this advice sounds familiar, that's because dealing with jet lag is very similar to what we do every day when we use light to reset our body clocks. It's what PMer chronotypes do in their day-to-day lives to combat social jet lag. Light is the tool we can best use every day in our lives to regulate our sleep-wake cycles, whether or not we ever fly long haul.

The Night Shift

Think of shift workers and you're likely to conjure up images of night shifts in a factory, doctors and nurses in a hospital, perhaps even bar staff, and the changing patterns of their work. But technology and the culture of working late into the night mean we're all guilty of pulling the occasional night shift.

I have worked with a professional poker player who spends his nights online in high-stakes games. There's a night shift that doesn't immediately spring to mind. He has to manage the challenges of a daytime family life in conjunction with his work, so in effect the challenge he faces is just the same as that of the doctor, nurse, or factory worker: how to manage a lifestyle that is completely at odds with our body clocks.

As we discussed all the way back in Chapter 1, being at war with our bodies in the long term can have serious repercussions, as Russell Foster, director of the Sleep and Circadian Neuroscience Institute at the University of Oxford, says: "Disrupted sleep, such as in shift workers, can lead to a multitude of problems ranging across suppressed immunity, greater risks of cancer, an increased risk of coronary heart disease and even metabolic disorders such as diabetes II."

If you're working at night, when your body naturally wants to produce melatonin and put you in a sleep state, you are bypassing the sleep window where urge and need collide. When you come home in the morning, with the sun up and your sleep pressure high but your circadian urge dipping, you are going to struggle to achieve the quality of sleep you would get at night. If we return to the circadian rhythms chart in Chapter 1, we can see the spectrum of functions your body naturally wants to do in harmony with the rising and setting of the sun. Working a night shift is certainly not on there.

When working nights, we effectively have to reset our body clock to work to the new time zone we find ourselves in, just as we would with jet lag. With the R90 program, we can look at using light in the form of daylight lamps and dawn simulators along with our windows of time—at night, the midday and early-evening slots, our ninety-minute breaks, and our pre- and post-sleep routines—to adjust to our new timetable. For PM chronotypes, this shift is obviously going to be easier.

So when we come home in the morning after a shift, we don't go right to bed. That's not what people working in the day do. Instead, we would come home, have a meal (if we *really* want to adjust to nights, this would be a traditional evening meal, not breakfast), and make this time our "evening." If you have children, you could spend some time with them before they go to school, maybe even do the school run, so you're not becoming completely alienated from the daytime hours and your family life.

If you don't have children, you could simply unwind as you would in the evening, perhaps watching some television or reading a book (though a glass of wine might feel a *little* inappropriate at 8 a.m.). Get your pre-sleep routine started ninety minutes before your targeted sleep time. It is here that blackout becomes even more important than it would at night. Just like a vampire, you need to keep the daylight out of your sleeping

A Night-Shift Worker's Five-Cycle Routine

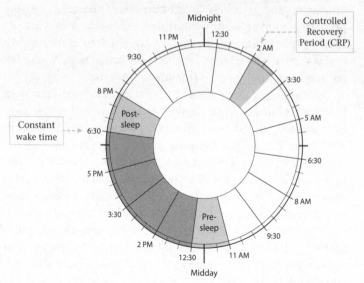

environment, and if possible, darken the room you're spending your pre-sleep routine in, so your body feels that night is falling.

When you are sleeping during the day, it's important to use the two CRP windows of midday (1–3 p.m.) and early evening (5–7 p.m.). Midday is especially important, as your circadian urge, mirroring the 2–3 a.m. period at night, is at its peak here. If you were able to, say, target a sleep time of 12:30 p.m., it would enable you to get to sleep and take advantage of this period. Getting five cycles in during the day is challenging, with broken sleep very common, but four from here, taking you through to 6:30 p.m., would allow you to use some of the early-evening slot.

The wake time in the evening should be constant too, and being woken with light is even more important than it is for a day worker. If your wake time is 6:30 p.m., that means it will be dark in winter, so you're going to need that light—get a dawn simulator. In summer, the bigger challenge is blocking the light out to sleep. As soon as you wake, get the blackout blinds or curtains open and get some daylight on you. Then go about your post-sleep routine: empty your bladder, fuel and hydrate, do some light exercise. Again, if you have children and/or a partner, you have a bit of time here to spend with them. You're not entirely alienating yourself from day-to-day life.

Once you get to work, light is vital. Standard artificial light is too weak, so you need daylight lamps if possible. Blue light isn't so badly timed here, as it helps with the suppression of melatonin. You want to be awake at this time, after all.

The obvious window for a CRP is around 2–3 a.m., the time of deepest sleepiness for those on a daytime schedule. Use this for a thirty- or (if your job allows) ninety-minute cycle. Caffeine can be a powerful performance enhancer for night-shift workers, but remember that the daily limit still applies: 400 milligrams, and don't forget the half-life of up to six hours. Shift workers are more likely to be at risk of obesity, so diet and exercise are important too.[11]

Stick to this every day and, as you trick your body clock into adjusting to a new sleep-wake cycle, you might just feel, as you would when you adjust to a new time zone, you've cracked it by the end of the week. However, for many shift workers, this is when they try to revert to daylight hours to reengage with family, friends, and social opportunities. Even worse, for those on ever-changing patterns of shifts, they are effectively constantly changing to different time zones, so they're always out of kilter with their surroundings.

Constantly making these adjustments is shown to have an impact on health. A study on more than seventy thousand night-shift-working female nurses over a twenty-two-year period showed that those working rotating night shifts for more than five years were more likely to die early, and more likely to do so through heart disease, while those working these shifts for over fifteen years had an increased chance of dying of lung cancer.[12]

This constant adjustment is clearly bad for our health, with those on rotating shifts demonstrating more problems than those who work nights permanently. While the R90 program can allow you to at least try to manage the difficulties inherent in shift work, in the long term there is a decision to be made: How long are you willing to keep on doing this? Five years? Ten? Your whole career? For many, there is little choice in the hours they work, but where there is the option, these are the kind of questions you will need to ask yourself sooner or later.

Even my client the professional poker player, who enjoys the benefits of working from home so that he can take a CRP at night when he wants (poker game permitting) and doesn't have to travel, will have to make a decision eventually, as cheating the clock will take its toll. It always does.

The War on Winter

At the start of the chapter Rebecca was trying a new wake time of 5 a.m. With spring on its way and the clocks going forward in most states on the second Sunday in March, the extra light and daylight hours would help Rebecca make this change more easily. But would she have been quite so enthusiastic about the idea if we had been talking in October, with winter on its way?

On the first Sunday of November every year, clocks in most states go back an hour (*spring* forward, *fall* back), which, along with the already encroaching darker nights that winter brings, means that the evenings become darker still. Daylight saving was first introduced during the First World War in an effort to conserve fuel in Germany, and Europe and the United States soon followed suit—though it didn't become a federal standard in the United States until the 1960s, in an effort to standardize time in the transportation industry. While daylight saving is not in effect from November through early March, there are plenty of supporters for the idea of remaining on this time all year round. A 2008 report from the US Department of Energy estimated that extending daylight saving by just four weeks would save about enough energy to power 100,000 homes for a year.[13] More than a dozen states have debated observing daylight-saving time year-round.[14] Meanwhile, in Britain, the Royal Society for the Prevention of Accidents (RoSPA) estimates that the lighter evenings "would have the net effect of saving around 80 lives and 212 serious injuries a year," and there would be an increase in leisure activities in the evening, helping to combat obesity, particularly in the young. It is also thought that seasonal affective disorder, which affects 1.6 billion people around the globe, is related to daylight-saving transitions and could be reduced by an extra hour of daylight.[15]

Seasonal affective disorder occurs when people with otherwise completely fine mental health suffer symptoms associated with depression at a regular, recurring period each year, usually winter. The truth is, almost all of us suffer some kind of what we like to call "the winter blues." Mood and motivation tend to drop in winter, it seems more difficult to get up in the morning, it's dark and cold (or at least cooler, even if you live in the southern United States), our eating habits can change to carbohydrate-heavy "comfort" foods instead of the fresh salads and light meals of summer, and, when we look to the animal kingdom, the idea of hibernation doesn't seem so bad. Indeed, many of us go through our own form of hibernation in the winter: going to work and coming home, staying in more in the evenings and on the weekends, doing less exercise because our mood and motivation are low. Television-viewing figures peak in the winter months.

Throughout my career in sports, I have yet to meet an athlete who isn't affected by this change in season. There is an urge to slow down in activity, just as there is for those staying in and watching more television at home, but in sports like football, basketball, and hockey, with regular seasons stretching from fall to winter and beyond, this simply isn't an option.

Aside from the cold weather, which can leave us unwilling commuters in the morning, the main obstacle we face in winter is the lack of light. Serotonin production can be disrupted, more melatonin might be produced, and our body clock, which depends on light to set it, can be affected, throwing our circadian rhythms out of whack.

Dark evenings are obviously a big part of this. Football players tend to train outdoors (though they spend plenty of time indoors in the gym too), so they will get some daylight during the day, but most of us work indoors. In the summer, this is OK because we go home in daylight and we can spend our evenings outdoors. But in winter we work all day indoors and then go home in the dark.

Getting out into the daylight in the morning, when we have breaks, and at lunchtime is essential at this time of year, even if it's cold outside. Invest in daylight products to help. I introduce daylight lamps at the soccer and rugby clubs I work with, and you can do the same in your home and office.

You are likely to feel more fatigued in the dark evenings when you get home from work, so use the early-evening slot for a CRP. Have a fifteen-minute blast on a daylight lamp, either during or after your CRP, to give you a boost so you can make more of your evening.

Pester your HR department at work to provide you with a daylight desk lamp if you struggle in winter. Your colleagues won't notice—they'll just assume it's another desk lamp—when you put it on during the midafternoon slump. Use your midday CRP. Your employer will enjoy the benefits of a happier, more productive employee.

Treat yourself to a product for your home, so you can enjoy the benefits of elevated mood and motivation, and you might find that reaching for the television remote isn't your first instinct in the evening—maybe you will make it to the gym or to meet your friends for dinner after all.

Heads Up

Hollywood superstar Will Smith, decked out in a gray suit and sporting a Nigerian accent in his role as Dr. Bennet Omalu in the movie *Concussion*, scribbles furiously on a whiteboard in an office with an audience of two other doctors. He describes the perils of a particular playing position with the objective logic his character's medical expertise brings to the table, rather than a fan's perspective: "It is an unremitting storm of subconcussive blows. The head as a weapon on every single play of every single game and every single practice from the time he was a little boy to a college man, culminating in an eighteen-year professional career. By my calculations, Mike Webster sustained more than seventy thousand blows to his head."

He talks of G-forces equivalent to the force of being hit on the head with a sledgehammer, and of Webster's brain being choked and leaving him unrecognizable, even to himself. In the dramatic climax to the scene, Will Smith looks to the camera and delivers his line: "I don't know football, I've never played, but I'm telling you, playing football killed Mike Webster."

Dr. Bennet Omalu is a Nigerian American pathologist who discovered chronic traumatic encephalopathy (CTE), a degenerative brain disease caused by repeated blows to the head, in the former NFL player Mike Webster, who had struggled with mental illness before his death.[16] While the NFL was slow to accept Omalu's findings—and both the film and the book on which it is based detail his struggle—in March 2016 it at last admitted a link between football and CTE. This could have huge ramifications not only for those retired from the game and playing now but also for the future of the sport, as parents already worried about the risk of physical injury now contemplate the very real threat of brain disease too for their children, the aspiring players of tomorrow.

Football isn't the only sport in which this is being taken seriously. Boxing is a sport in which repeated blows to the head are almost the whole point of it—the aptly named dementia pugilistica, a type of CTE, was recognized long before Omalu's discovery—and in the game of rugby, the nearest equivalent Britain has to American football, concussion and head injury issues are a hot topic. And this is partly why I'm getting involved in this sport.

I have worked with clubs and player welfare organizations in both codes of professional rugby in the United Kingdom, union and league. With the latter, I was contracted to coach all the players throughout the Super League, while in union I have done likewise with several clubs and the Rugby Players' Association, as well as working with the English national team, including advising them on recovery strategies during their tour of Australia in 2016, in which they made history by winning a series there for the first time.

While "the head as a weapon" isn't part of the game in the same way it is in the NFL, the collisions and the risk of head injuries and concussion very much are. As advances in sports continue and the players use these gains to become quicker, fitter, and stronger, the hits just keep getting harder.

Rugby union player Alex Corbisiero, who took a year out of the game in 2016 during what should have been his peak years as a player, told the *Guardian* newspaper, "I was physically and mentally spent after ten years of full-time rugby. The intensity, the physicality, the injuries and the pressure I put on myself took its toll. I knew if I wanted to play rugby again I had to stop for a while."

As is so common in modern professional sports, the schedules in the game are incredibly demanding, with many feeling that too many games are being packed into too tight a time frame, without the necessary scope for recovery. As Christian Day, the Rugby Players' Association chairman, puts it, "Sooner or later, someone needs to say, 'Look, we're going to destroy these guys.' They're going to retire by the time they're thirty years old; they're not going to be able to walk by the age of forty-five. I just hope someone at the top of the game is planning."

I can't change the nature of their sport—that is up to the administrators in the game, and, just as the NFL found, it is no easy feat when sponsorship and broadcast deals are involved. So while their playing and training schedules remain packed, and while the hits just keep coming at such a ferocious intensity, all I can do is show the players the R90 program and educate them on how they can manage their lives to recover more efficiently so that they're not doing too much to exacerbate the problem. When it comes to the potential for long-term mental and physical repercussions from the sport, aggregating as many marginal gains as possible in taking care of their bodies and minds is all the players can really do to defend themselves, short of following Corbisiero's lead and taking a sabbatical, which simply isn't an option for most. It's a short career, after all.

While cracking heads isn't a workplace health risk for many of us, the mental side of things very much is. Stress, burnout, depression, and anxiety are issues many of us face or might have experienced thanks to the frenetic pace of our lives, and diseases like Alzheimer's and dementia might be awaiting some of us further down the line, just like CTE for football players, if we don't reform our approach to recovery.

Sleep and mental illness are inextricably linked. Depression and anxiety disorders include an element of sleep disruption—as do psychiatric illnesses like bipolar disorder and schizophrenia—and while professional athletes are fortunate in many respects that they often have first-rate medical staff on hand to turn to and to keep an eye on them, the sad fact is that there is still a great deal of stigma attached to admitting to mental health problems in sports and in society as a whole. Performers often hide their issues and struggle on, just as many people do in their jobs every day, without seeking the help they need.

While I can help a person manage their disrupted sleep through periods of anxiety and stress, when it comes to things like depression and mental illness, the right kind of medical help is required. Treating patients is, after all, what the clinical approach is for.

In many ways, our modern working practices can be traced back to the invention of the lightbulb, which opened up the night to us. Now we're in need of another light-bulb moment to redefine our approach to work and rest. Companies like Google are leading the way in well-being reforms and flexible work hours, but not all of us are lucky enough to work for such organizations, and that is why taking responsibility yourself and adopting the R90 program is so important if you want to manage the increasing demands of today's world—and look after yourself in anticipation of tomorrow's.

TEN

The Home Team

Sex, Partners, and the Modern Family

The first time I went into Arsenal soccer club in London, it was to address the whole squad about sleep and recovery. I had met Gary Lewin, the club's physiotherapist, through working with the English national team, and he had recommended me to the manager, Arsène Wenger.

While my involvement with Manchester United had happened quite organically and informally, with Alex Ferguson's openness to my speculative letter allowing me to help Gary Pallister out originally and then grow my role to work with the rest of the squad, I hadn't really thought too much about where it was leading. But as I traveled down to London in an official capacity it clicked that I was about to become a sleep coach to the two biggest soccer clubs in England, as well as the national team. As I was really only at the beginning of my career in sports, with so much still to learn, the realization was an exciting one—but it made me a little nervous too, so I took my son James with me for support.

In a conference room in the club's training ground at London Colney, near St. Albans in Hertfordshire, in front of the whole first-team squad, Gary Lewin introduced me. I started my presentation, explaining to the players the techniques and relevant aspects of sleep that, although still raw, were the beginnings of the R90 program. About halfway through, I was demonstrating some products when a couple of the young players asked if they could try one of the sleeping surfaces.

"Sure," I said.

They must have thought, *We're going to have some fun with this*. They both proceeded to get on the sleeping surface . . . and then they started messing around like guys do, making almost everyone in the room erupt into laughter. My presentation threatened to descend into chaos, until a player stood up and said, "That's enough!"

Everyone in the room stopped and looked toward him. "We're here to listen," he said, "so let's keep it quiet."

It was Thierry Henry, who would one day go on to play for the New York Red Bulls. Thank you, Thierry.

Sex Before the Big Game

Boxers might be warned to abstain the night before a fight, soccer players before the match, and a sprinter before the race, but there is conflicting evidence as to whether sex will inhibit performance. For some athletes it might even help. Do *you* abstain the night before a big event in your life?

This was something that always fascinated a close friend and colleague of mine, Nick Broad.[1] He was head of sports science at Chelsea Football Club, and he believed that sex could be used very effectively for a player with the right (personal) approach.

Good sex is an incredibly pleasurable and powerful way to reduce stress, anxiety, and worry. It allows our minds to focus on an exciting and spontaneous action, losing ourselves in the moment. It can make us feel loved, wanted, and secure. It's a natural form of exercise—the more regular, the better—and its afterglow can provide a warm, relaxing sense of well-being. And, particularly for men, it seems to be the perfect platform to send some of us right off to sleep.

Put like this, sex sounds like a pre-sleep routine we can all get on board with. But the idea of using it as any kind of routine is about as big a passion-killer as there is. Your bed is for sleeping first, and sex a close second, so don't just confine your sex life exclusively to the bed. Use your imagination, keep things fresh and exciting, and allow your mind to make its strongest association between the bed and sleep. You can have sex anywhere (as long as it won't land you in trouble).

Sex isn't always good either. One person in the couple may not always be in the mood, which can inspire feelings of rejection or pressure to perform, or one may be left dissatisfied by the end while the other drifts off carefree into sleep. Partners can be left anxious, unhappy, and drained by sex, and it can take a toll on a relationship.

Then there is the question of sex being physically draining. Unless you're indulging in several hours of bedroom gymnastics that interfere with your targeted sleep cycles, it's unlikely to have much of a physical impact. Clemens Westerhof, a Dutchman who achieved some success managing Nigeria's soccer team, put it best when he said, "It's not the sex which tires out young players. It's the staying up all night looking for it."

Perhaps the best question any of us should ask ourselves the night before a big event is what the effect is likely to be on us. If it's good sex, with the stress-busting, mood-boosting, and relaxing benefits, then it is likely to give us some escape from the worries of the next day's event and help put us in a better position to sleep and wake up revitalized. If it's the bad kind, however, with anxiety keeping us up into the night, then it's surely better to stick to the "no sex before the big game" rule.

Perhaps the last word on the subject should come from someone with a broader sample size than many clinical trials are capable of producing—the legendary Manchester United soccer star George Best. "I certainly never found it had any effect on my performance," he once said. "Maybe best not the hour before, but the night before makes no odds."

Do You Come Here Often?

Where athletes will differ from the rest of us mere mortals after they've had sex the night before the big event is that, instead of turning over and going to sleep, they will get up and retire to a different room to spend the night in their personal single-size sleep kit. Sex before a big game is all well and good, but compromising on recovery by having a partner lying next to you? Not an option even worth contemplating for many elite athletes. It's all about recovery risk-management to them.

The role a regular partner can play in our sleep is huge. When we address each of the Key Sleep Recovery Indicators, we're initially doing it only with ourselves in mind. But when I'm working with someone like Rebecca at the start of Chapter 9, whose partner is sleeping on the sofa bed while she tries to regain some control over her sleep, I know that once she has achieved a kind of stability in her own routine on the blank canvas that is just her in the bed, I'm going to have to do a sleep profile with her partner, because who knows what they might be bringing back into the recovery room to cause problems.

In a survey, 17 percent of women and 5 percent of men reported that partner disturbance had affected their own sleep.[2] Snoring, apnea (it's usually a partner who notices this), blanket hogging, getting up in the night, and fidgeting are all factors that a partner could be bringing to bed with them. But there are more subtle issues at play too that we might not have even considered before that can have an impact, such as different sleep and wake times. Getting into bed when a partner is already in there asleep can disturb them, just as the earlier riser can disrupt the sleep of the partner trying to sleep in later.

"Are you left- or right-handed?" is a pickup line unlikely to rival "Do you come here often?" for popularity anytime soon, but it will certainly have a big effect on your sleep if the relationship goes anywhere. When we fall asleep facing someone or spooning with them, no matter how loved-up we are, one of us will eventually "blink" first and turn away from the other into our own personal space. We won't even remember doing it, but breathing in someone else's air is a disturbance, and we will move away intuitively.

Sleeping with someone has pre- and post-sleep benefits, but in an ideal world we would pre-sleep together, then go into our own individual sleep rooms, where we'd sleep undisturbed. Then we'd get up and enjoy post-sleep fully recovered and happy to engage with our partners and our day. Sleeping separately is natural for us—we do it throughout our formative years. Perhaps the bedrooms of the future might include such a feature.

Our ideal sleeping position is fetal, lying on the nondominant side (right-handers sleep on their left side and vice versa), which achieves the psychological reassurance of protecting the heart, organs, and genitals with the stronger side. If you sleep alone, it doesn't matter where you sleep in the bed, but once a partner is involved it becomes more complicated. There is clearly a preferred side of the bed. If you stand at the foot of the bed, looking up toward it, then the right-hand side of the bed is the preferred position for the right-hander, and the left-hand side for the southpaw.

In these positions, both people are lying on the correct side of their body for sleep, and facing away from their partner, out into clear space, so there is no obstacle in front of them to disturb them. If you're a left-hander and your partner is right-handed, you are made for each other in this sense.

But if both partners in the bed are either right- or left-handed, then one person is going to be sleeping on the wrong side of the bed for them. The right-hander on the left side or the left-hander on the right side will be facing *into* the bed and into

The Perfect Match: Left- and Right-Handed Partners
Sleeping on Correct Sides of the Bed

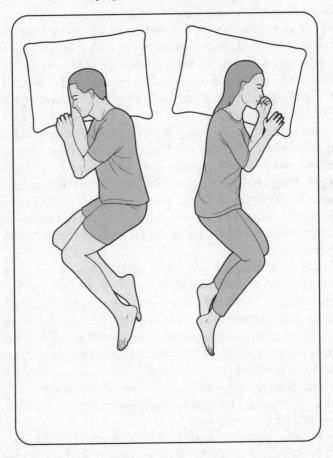

their partner's back, exposing them to the possibility of more disturbance. And if they face out of the bed—if, for example, they "blink" first, having fallen asleep in a romantic embrace— they are sleeping on their dominant side. The non-dominant side of our body is less sensitive, so it's easier for it to be in the same position all night throughout sleep.

So what's the solution—trade in your partner for a more suitable one? Love is blind, so they say, and it certainly doesn't pay heed to our dominant sides. Instead, be aware of which of you is sleeping on their wrong side and try to make things easier for that person. The biggest bed your recovery room can hold is paramount here (a king is simply the *minimum* size for two adults), and if you toss and turn or get up during the night, be aware that your partner is likely to be facing toward you, and you're more likely to disturb them.

Understanding just how much we can disturb our partner's sleep allows us to adopt new philosophies when we're doing things like looking at a new house to buy or rent. We prioritize the master bedroom size, making sure it will fit a king bed. I've cooked in kitchens of all shapes and sizes and showered in small bathrooms, but with a partner in my life I need a bedroom that will hold a bed big enough for two adults to share.

When a big event is on the horizon—the marathon or triathlon you're training for, the project you're preparing, or even the baby you're expecting—you can also do what the athletes do and take your partner out of the equation. Move to the spare room or set up a temporary bed—an air bed, foam pad, or sofa bed—in the living room. Pregnancy, particularly in the later stages, can cause a great deal of disturbance to a woman's sleep, as she struggles to make herself comfortable during the night, and it can be beneficial for both the expectant mother and her partner to sleep separately. A king might be a bed for two people—but three can be a crowd at this time.

When Roger Federer plays at Wimbledon it has been reported that he rents two houses next door to each other: one for his wife and children, and the other for his staff. He doesn't sleep in the family house. The athletes I worked with prior to the Olympic Games in Rio in 2016 had their own portable R90 sleep kits, so they had a single-sleeping option.

In this sense the bed becomes a kind of sanctuary for a couple to relax in, have sex in if they like, but at that moment when they turn over and go to sleep, the athlete gets out and retires to their sleep kit. It reduces the amount of potential disturbance to just what you bring to bed yourself, a marginal-gains approach to your event—and your relationship. So next time you read about a celebrity couple or hear about your friends sleeping in separate beds, don't be so quick to judge. They might just be reaping the benefits of getting the best sleep possible, waking up refreshed and in a great mood, with their relationship stronger than ever.

The Family Way

When we're expecting a child, modern medical technology can tell us all sorts of things, such as the sex and the potential for complications, conditions, or disability—but it still can't tell us what the baby is really going to be like. I have raised two children of my own, one of whom slept all the time and the other who screamed for three years straight—or at least that's what it felt like.

If you've been applying the R90 program to your lives, use a correctly profiled sleep kit in the right recovery room, have your constant wake time, know how to use CRPs, and work in harmony with your circadian rhythms, chronotype, and sleep cycles, then you have a good deal of preparation work already in place to deal with the disruption a newborn can potentially cause to your life. At least that's the theory.

You have your twenty-four-hour schedule anchored around your constant wake time, and you should stick to this wake time where possible. You have your midday and early-evening CRP windows, and you have your ninety-minute intervals of targeted sleep times at night. Once the baby arrives, the mother moves to a schedule based entirely around the baby's, which essentially consists of sleep, wake, feed, and bowel and bladder movements on repeat. The partner needs to share in this as much as possible; otherwise it can put extra pressures on the relationship, though the mother is biologically predisposed to waking at the sound of her baby's cry.

So, with a constant wake time of 6:30 a.m. and a newborn waking at 2 a.m., you would get up, see to the baby, and, assuming you get him or her back to sleep, you now look at your sleep times instead of just going straight back to bed. If you've been a parent, you might well have experienced the feeling of going back to bed and finding you can't sleep, maybe getting frustrated because you're so exhausted from it all. Don't waste your valuable time on this. If it's 2:30 a.m., you target a 3:30 a.m. sleep time, so you do some pre-sleep-style activities—declutter, do a bit of housework, meditate, or even watch a bit of television—before you sleep. If you're lucky enough to sleep until your alarm sounds, you get up at your usual wake time.

Don't sleep during the day outside of the CRP windows if you can help it. If the baby goes to sleep at 1 p.m., do likewise—get a thirty- or ninety-minute cycle in. But don't have two or three cycles just because the baby does too. You don't want to fight your body clock. Get up, do some positive things to catch up—laundry is a constant with a newborn, so put a load in the washing machine, or tidy up, or do a little something for yourself before the baby wakes up again.

Eventually, if you're lucky, the baby will develop patterns, and you can start to move your R90 program in accordance with this, try to slot in with their routine. You've got some control of your recovery during this period, while many other new parents are just floundering around and nodding off indiscriminately, lying in bed struggling to sleep at night and feeling like everything is out of their hands. There are plenty of books and advice forums telling you about what to do and look out for in terms of the baby, but not so much telling you how to take care of yourself. With your R90 program, you can take control.

And if you're not lucky? That's OK too. I've experienced it both ways. If you're repeatedly up during the night, sleep-deprived to what feels like the point of mania, and finding yourself saying things in anger to your partner that you would never have dreamed of before, it's nothing that other parents haven't been through. Think of yourself in terms of the round-the-world sailor, getting by on thirty minutes' sleep every twelve hours. Think of those who adopt the Uberman sleep schedule, in which extreme polyphasic sleepers have a twenty-minute nap every four hours—only two hours of sleep in total per day.

We are incredibly robust creatures when it comes to dealing with lack of sleep, and, unlike many of the things we do today that deprive us of sleep, evolution has hardwired us to cope with raising a child. Try your best to keep in harmony with your R90 program, try to maintain a reasonable diet and look after yourself, even if that just means little breaks here and there, in tandem with your partner, and don't be too hard on yourself or your partner when you can't stick to the R90 or when you're operating on only a couple of cycles a night. It isn't forever. It will get easier as they get older.

"Lazy" Teenagers

Children grow up. Newborns soon develop their own circadian rhythms and adjust to the light-dark cycle (it's just dark in the womb). The National Sleep Foundation recommends fourteen to seventeen hours of sleep per day for a newborn, but this amount decreases as they get older, with nine to eleven hours the recommendation by the time they start school and, once they hit fourteen, eight to ten hours.

Taking your own sleep seriously is, ultimately, an informed decision of your own to make. You can read this book, make up your mind about what you take from it, and hopefully apply as much as you can to your own life. When it comes to children, however, there isn't a decision to be made: you *must* take their sleep seriously.

Sleep is vital for a child's development. Their body and mind need plenty of it to grow properly. Ensuring they have the right quantity *and* quality of sleep involves introducing some of the measures we've talked about so far—such as providing a suitable sleeping environment and some kind of pre- and post-sleep routines, which they will come to associate with going to sleep and starting the day, and making sure they're not overstimulating (on sugar, in this case, since caffeine is less of a consideration for kids)—as well as some that don't apply quite so much to adults, such as a regular sleep time.

The R90 is a great way to ensure that you can adjust your sleep and wake times to fit into the hours your children require. It provides confidence and flexibility if circumstances dictate a change, and it helps engage parents and children together in becoming more sleep aware. Spot your child's chronotype early so that when they are at school they know when their best time to study is, an empowering piece of awareness to take through their education and then into the workplace. If your children grow into being sports fans you can even tell them you take tips from the sports sleep coach—who shows the stars how to do it.

However, the R90 program is not for children to use. Don't try to limit or restrict their time; just put everything in place for them to be able to get plenty of good-quality sleep with as little interference as possible, and let them do their thing with what comes naturally. Most children are good sleepers, and you can educate them about everything you've put in place to help them when they get older.

Once they reach adolescence, things get more complicated. Teenagers still need a lot of sleep, particularly because during sleep they release the hormone that produces the growth spurt they experience during this time. Unfortunately, getting enough sleep is complicated by biological factors—and increasingly by social and technology temptations.

No matter what their chronotype is before adolescence, when they reach puberty the biological changes in their bodies cause their circadian rhythms to shift. They start producing melatonin later at night, and so they naturally want to go to bed later and, given that they need more sleep than an adult, they will want to sleep in the following morning. It's time to cut teenagers some slack—they sleep in because that's what their bodies want them to do.

However, an early start at school or college gets in the way of that. The school timetable conflicts with a teenager's natural rhythms. A 2008 study comparing sleeping habits in students on school days and on vacation showed that "with the impact of school schedule, students accrued a significant sleep debt, obtaining insufficient sleep for their needs and reporting lowered mood and daytime functioning."[3] The students were, of course, sleeping in on the weekend.

This delaying of the body clock is exacerbated by the social opportunities that open up for teenagers. Many of them want to be out later with their friends in the evening, not cooped up at home. Any parent who has raised a child through adolescence will be familiar with this, but it's only those doing it now or in recent times who will be familiar with the added problems technology poses.

Even if a teenager goes to their room at a reasonable hour, the multitude of options technology presents them with means they might decide to play video games or engage with social media on their devices late into the night. We have already discussed the impact blue light exposure from this technology can have, potentially suppressing melatonin production and making it harder to go to sleep, but there is also the addictive nature of video games and social media to take into account. If a teenager isn't sleepy because of their shifted rhythms, saving the world and blowing up bad guys in a video game is an enticing entertainment option, but with the heightened alertness and adrenaline they will experience from playing it keeping them up even longer and ensuring that when the alarm goes off in the morning for school, possibly after they've fallen asleep with the technology still on, they are not going to be at their best for their morning classes.

This is the "junk sleep" that Idzikowski talks about, in which neither the quality nor the duration of sleep required is achieved. In adolescents this can severely stymie their development and education, can affect their mood and concentration, and could have a long-term impact on their health (mental and physical) and weight.

An Australian study published in the *Journal of Adolescent Health* in 2016 concluded that "video games and online social media were risk factors for shorter and poorer sleep, whereas time with family was protective of sleep duration."[4] If only the answer was as simple as to tell adolescents to turn off the tech and spend more time with the family. While it is unfair to tar all teenagers with the same brush, as many will heed the advice and be aware of the damage it could be having on their education and development, those of us who have raised teenagers or indeed remember being teenagers ourselves will know that, quite often, any such well-meaning advice from a parent can fall on deaf ears. However, a parent should attempt to find some way to manage an adolescent's tech use before sleep, whether that's through agreeing to a deal whereby they don't play their video games after a certain time at night or removing the technology from the bedroom altogether. Asking a teenager to hand over their smartphone, however, might be a trickier proposition, so good luck with that.

Adolescents simply aren't getting enough sleep on school nights, and the perfect storm of their hormonally shifted rhythms, social opportunities, and technology alongside the time school starts is to blame. So what if we were able to allow teenagers more time in bed on a school-day morning?

Moving high school and college start times for teenagers to 10 a.m. would provide a timetable with the needs of the students in mind rather than those of parents and teachers. No more 9 a.m. classes or exams would mean that teenagers would no longer be expected to perform at a time that was at odds with their body clocks, and it would cut down their sleep deprivation too.

Tomorrow's First Team

I work with a lot of teenagers in the sporting world: the potential Olympians of tomorrow and the youth squads and young players at soccer clubs in particular. I see firsthand the impact their shifted body clocks and technology have on them, and it is around this age, in the mid-teens, with the demands of their sport and lifestyle making time a precious commodity to them, that they can start using the R90 program, albeit in a format that looks at six cycles rather than five as ideal.

A swimming star of the future has to be at school at 8 a.m. just like any other teenager, but they have to fit in their hours at the pool either before or after school. How is that impacting their need for a good amount of sleep for their development and recovery every day? Starting school at 10 a.m. would give them more leeway; changing the clocks to remain on summer time all year round would give them lighter evenings after school in the winter. It's not just athletes who would benefit: young people are generally more likely to do leisure activities when it's light.

At the academies of soccer clubs in the United Kingdom I see teenagers from all walks of life. Some of them don't have the parental figures at home to instill discipline about sleep and recovery, and to explain to them how, if they want a good future in the game, they need it even more than those playing on the first team. They're up late at night, playing video games, hanging out with their friends, and certainly not sleeping for six cycles at night. It's going to have serious consequences if they don't work it out. With the R90 program, they can use a redefined approach to sleep in today's world, using technology as a positive tool and seeing a way to recover that can be flexible and engaging for them. It's up to me to really get through to them and instill some trust in them—and it's up to them to be disciplined about it too, because ultimately it's about developing the tools to manage your recovery yourself.

Top soccer stars are often accused of living in a bubble, up in their ivory towers, but what choice do they really have? Whereas once a player would have to keep an eye out for the paparazzi if they were on vacation or having an evening out, now, thanks to the cameras on our phones, *everyone* is a potential paparazzo. Sports figures are paranoid and cut off because they have to be—they can't afford to put a foot out of line in public. I've seen the toll this can take on young players struggling to adjust to it. Some of them can't manage it. *Awww, you might think, they get paid well enough to put up with it.* But money doesn't give you immunity from depression and anxiety disorders.

Technology has created a bubble for normal teenagers to live in too, doing much of their social interaction on their phones indoors at home. I've known teenagers who do not have a clue as to which shops are in their town because they don't need to—they can get everything they need brought to their lap from their phone. That includes knowledge, which must leave some of them wondering, *What do we need school and teachers for?*

The changes technology has brought to our society have brought with them huge benefits, but we need to be careful with it, especially as regards young people. A Microsoft Consumer Insights report in Canada claimed that the average human attention span decreased from twelve seconds in 2000 to eight seconds in 2013. Of the eighteen- to twenty-four-year-old Canadians they questioned, 77 percent said that they reach for their phone when nothing else is occupying their attention, and 73 percent said that the last thing they do before going to bed at night is check their phone.

We haven't seen any clinical data about the long-term effects of a lifetime of this kind of technology use because we haven't yet had it for the long term. The generations growing up now will be the first to have this for a lifetime, and we can already see the impact it is having on their sleep. As parents, we must do what we can to limit its use—just as we should try to do the same in our own lives.

I have universities and schools getting in touch with me now, asking me to come in and speak to students, because they are starting to see there's a problem. They want to do something about it.

With Southampton Football Club, I helped implement a top-down scheme in which everyone from the manager and his staff down to the youth squad took part in the program.

Club doctor Steve Baynes, who is a former Team Sky doctor, instigated the project, which continues today, even though the managers change. Southampton has a proven track record of producing talented young players through their youth system who go on to play on the first team, often for their national teams, and sometimes they continue on to play for the biggest clubs in the world. Real Madrid and Wales star Gareth Bale is one such product of Southampton's youth system.

Southampton is a club that takes the future of their young people very seriously indeed. If we want to produce the engineers, athletes, scientists, writers, and other great talents of tomorrow, we need to do likewise and start taking seriously the rest and recovery of our young people.

Your Personal Best

Standing with my son James and my family in the crowd in the Estádio da Luz in Lisbon, watching England play France at the 2004 European Championship football tournament, was a wonderful moment for me. England was playing well and winning 1–0, the atmosphere was electric, my family was next to me, and I'd contributed in my own way to it all—I'd worked with the squad and all the players had slept on my kit. It was just as if I'd been tucking the players in at night, as the media might once have said.

What does pride come before? By the end of the match, France's captain and star player, Zinedine Zidane, had scored two late goals to win the game and spoil the party. Same old England. But for a moment there—wow . . .

Only a few years after I'd first asked the question of Alex Ferguson and, by association, the whole world of sports, I'd found myself in a place I could never have imagined. Asking that question changed my career and it certainly changed my life, and I have been privileged to help change the lives of others as I've done so.

In the years after 2004 I would continue to ask the question, and work with exceptional athletes across all sports, from cycling to football and everything in between, as well as with tomorrow's star performers.

I'm still asking the question now—still knocking on doors and trying to find answers. It's why athletes and teams looking for the ultimate legal performance enhancer are getting in touch. It's why schools and universities, big business and ordinary people who want to change their lives are calling me. It's why I'm having conversations with people like Arianna Huffington, founder of the *Huffington Post* and leader of her own sleep revolution, and why I'm being invited to speak at former New York mayor Michael Bloomberg's global summit for leaders of major cities. Because they're all asking the question now, and you should be too: *What are we doing about our sleep?*

What are we doing about this process of mental and physical recovery? How are we going to change our approach to something we can no longer afford to take for granted? The potential consequences are severe and potentially fatal—cancer, obesity, diabetes, heart disease—and capable of casting you as a shadow of your former self in the form of depression, anxiety, burnout, and Alzheimer's. Depression kills, particularly in young men—the kind I see in sports academies across the United Kingdom and all over the world.

It doesn't have to be this way. With the R90 program you can redefine your approach to sleep just like the athletes and teams I work with, who bring home trophies and gold medals. You will see your mood, motivation, creativity, memory, energy levels, and alertness skyrocket. Your work, relationships, and family life will be enriched beyond measure because you'll be setting your own personal bests, time and time again.

It starts with you, but this is a team sport. You must then ask the question of your family, your children, your workplace, and your friends. Together, we can make it a huge cultural shift, a redefined approach so that the process of recovery joins exercise and diet as a three-pronged assault on bad living.

Forget about sleep as you knew it. The process of recovery is on a twenty-four-hour ticking clock, a constant rhythm that we all need to learn to groove with. Starting today doesn't mean when you go to bed tonight. It means right now.

So what are you waiting for?

Notes

Introduction: Don't Waste Your Valuable Time Sleeping

1. O. M. Buxton, S. W. Cain, S. P. O'Connor, J. H. Porter, J. F. Duffy, W. Wang, C. A. Czeisler, S. A. Shea, "Adverse Metabolic Consequences in Humans of Prolonged Sleep Restriction Combined with Circadian Disruption," *Science Translational Medicine*, April 11, 2012.

2. L. Xie, H. Kang, Q. Xu, M. J. Chen, Y. Liao, M. Thiyagarajan, J. O'Donnell, D. J. Christensen, C. Nicholson, J. J. Iliff, T. Takano, R. Deane, M. Nedergaard, "Sleep Drives Metabolite Clearance from the Adult Brain," *Science*, October 18, 2013.

3. UK Sleep Council statistics.

1. The Clock Is Ticking: Circadian Rhythms

1. J. M. Jones, "In U.S., 40% Get Less Than Recommended Amount of Sleep," Gallup, December 19, 2013.

2. Sleep Council, *The Great British Bedtime Report*, 2013, 3; National Sleep Foundation International Bedroom Poll, 2013.

3. American Psychological Association, "Stress and Sleep," press release, 2013.

4. S. A. Rahman, E. E. Flynn-Evans, D. Aeschbach, G. C. Brainard, C. A. Czeisler, S. W. Lockley, "Diurnal Spectral Sensitivity of the Acute Alerting Effects of Light," *Sleep* 37, no. 2 (February 2014): 271–81.

2. Running Fast and Slow: Chronotype

1. Munich Chronotype Questionnaire, University of Munich, https://www.bioinfo.mpg.de/mctq/core_work_life/core/introduction.jsp.

2. T. Roenneberg, T. Kuehnle, P. P. Pramstaller, J. Ricken, M. Havel, A. Guth, M. Merrow, "A Marker for the End of Adolescence," *Current Biology* 14, no. 24 (December 29, 2004).

3. D. H. Pesta, S. S. Angadi, M. Burtscher, C. K. Roberts, "The Effects of Caffeine, Nicotine, Ethanol, and Tetrahydrocannabinol on Exercise Performance," *Nutrition and Metabolism* 10, no. 1 (December 2013): 71.

4. M. S. Ganio, J. F. Klau, D. J. Casa, L. E. Armstrong, C. M. Maresh, "Effect of Caffeine on Sport-Specific Endurance Performance: A Systematic Review," *Journal of Strength and Conditioning Research* 23, no. 1 (January 2009): 315–24.

3. A Game of Ninety Minutes: Sleeping in Cycles, Not Hours

1. M. P. Walker, T. Brakefield, A. Morgan, J. A. Hobson, R. Stickgold, "Practice with Sleep Makes Perfect: Sleep-Dependent Motor Skill Learning," *Neuron* 35, no. 1 (July 3, 2002): 205–11.

2. E. Van Cauter, L. Plat, "Physiology of Growth Hormone Secretion During Sleep," *Journal of Pediatrics* 128, no. 5, part 2 (May 1996): 532–37.

3. D. J. Cai, S. A. Mednick, E. M. Harrison, J. C. Kanady, S. C. Mednick, "REM, Not Incubation, Improves Creativity by Priming Associative Networks," *Proceedings of the National Academy of Sciences of the United States of America* 106, no. 25 (June 23, 2009): 30–34.

4. T. Endo, C. Roth, H. P. Landolt, E. Werth, D. Aeschbach, P. Achermann, A. A. Borbély, "Selective REM Sleep Deprivation in Humans: Effects on Sleep and Sleep EEG," *American Journal of Physiology* 274, no. 4, part 2 (1998): R1186–94.

4. Warming Up and Cooling Down: Pre- and Post-Sleep Routines

1. American Psychological Association, "Stress and Sleep," press release, 2013.

2. M. P. Walker, "Sleep-Dependent Memory Processing," *Harvard Review of Psychology* 16, no. 5 (September–October 2008): 287–98.

3. "Latest Telecommuting Statistics," GlobalWorkplaceAnalytics.com, http://globalworkplaceanalytics.com/telecommuting-statistics, updated January 2016.

5. Time Out! Redefining Naps: Activity and Recovery Harmony

1. J. Warren, "How to Sleep Like a Hunter-Gatherer," *Discover*, December 2007.

2. O. Lahl, C. Wispel, B. Willigens, R. Pietrowsky, "An Ultra Short Episode of Sleep Is Sufficient to Promote Declarative Memory Performance," *Journal of Sleep Research* 17, no. 1 (March 2008): 3–10.

3. M. R. Rosekind, R. M. Smith, D. L. Miller, E. L. Co, K. B. Gregory, L. L. Webbon, P. H. Gander, J. V. Lebacqz, "Alertness Management: Strategic Naps in Operational Settings," *Journal of Sleep Research* 4, no. S2 (December 1995): 62–66.

4. M. Calabresi, "Air Traffic Controllers: Let Them Nap," *Time*, April 26, 2011.

5. A. Brooks, L. Lack, "A Brief Afternoon Nap Following Nocturnal Sleep Restriction: Which Nap Duration Is Most Recuperative?," *Sleep* 29, no. 6 (June 2006): 831–40.

6. K. A. Ericsson, N. Charness, P. J. Feltovich, R. R. Hoffman, *The Cambridge Handbook of Expertise and Expert Performance* (Cambridge: Cambridge University Press, 2006).

7. UK Department for Transport, "Sleep-Related Crashes on Sections of Different Road Types in the UK (1995–2001)," 2004.

8. National Highway Traffic Safety Administration, "Drowsy Driving," https://www.nhtsa.gov/risky-driving/drowsy-driving, accessed June 2017.

9. Federal Motor Carrier Safety Administration, US Department of Transportation, "Advanced Driver Fatigue Research," 2007.

10. Ericsson et al., *Cambridge Handbook of Expertise and Expert Performance*.

7. Recovery Room: The Sleeping Environment

1. A. Thompson, H. Jones, W. Gregson, G. Atkinson, "Effects of Dawn Simulation on Markers of Sleep Inertia and Post-Waking Performance in Humans," *European Journal of Applied Physiology* 114, no. 5 (May 2014): 1049–56; V. Gabel, M. Maire, C. F. Reichert, S. L. Chellappa, C. Schmidt, V. Hommes, A. U. Viola, C. Cajochen, "Effects of Artificial Dawn and Morning Blue Light on Daytime Cognitive Performance, Well-Being, Cortisol and Melatonin Levels," *Chronobiology International* 30, no. 8 (October 2013): 988–97.

2. Ofcom Communications Market Report, 2011.

8. A Head Start: Using Your R90 Recovery Program

1. R. H. Eckel, J. M. Jakicic, J. D. Ard, J. M. de Jesus, N. Houston Miller, V. S. Hubbard, I. M. Lee, A. H. Lichtenstein, C. M. Loria, B. E. Millen, C. A. Nonas, F. M. Sacks, S. C. Smith Jr., L. P. Svetkey, T. A. Wadden, S. Z. Yanovski, "2013 AHA/ACC Guideline on Lifestyle Management to Reduce Cardiovascular Risk: A Report of the

American College of Cardiology/American Heart Association Task Force on Practice Guidelines," *Journal of the American College of Cardiology* 63, no. 25, pt. B (July 1, 2014): 2960–84.

2. F. P. Cappuccio, D. Cooper, L. D'Elia, P. Strazzullo, M. A. Miller, "Sleep Duration Predicts Cardiovascular Outcomes: A Systematic Review and Meta-Analysis of Prospective Studies," *European Heart Journal*, February 7, 2011.

3. G. Howatson, P. G Bell, J. Tallent, B. Middleton, M. P. McHugh, J. Ellis, "Effect of Tart Cherry Juice (*Prunus cerasus*) on Melatonin Levels and Enhanced Sleep Quality," *European Journal of Nutrition* 51, no. 8 (December 2012): 909–16.

4. P. D. Loprinzi, B. J. Cardinal, "Association Between Objectively-Measured Physical Activity and Sleep," *Mental Health and Physical Activity*, December 2011.

5. "Total Number of Memberships at Fitness Centers/Health Clubs in the U.S. from 2000 to 2015 (in Millions)," Statista.com, https://www.statista.com/statistics/236123/us-fitness-center—health-club-memberships, accessed May 2017.

6. Parks Associates figures.

9. Sleeping with the Enemy: Sleep Problems

1. Rebecca is not her real name, and I have altered identifying elements. All my clients remain anonymous and their details confidential.

2. Chris Idzikowski, *Sound Asleep: The Expert Guide to Sleeping Well* (London: Watkins, 2013).

3. Persistence Market Research, "Global Market Study on Sleep Aids," July 2015.

4. US National Center for Health Statistics.

5. N. Gunja, "In the Zzz Zone: The Effects of Z-Drugs on Human Performance and Driving," *Journal of Medical Toxicology* 9, no. 2 (June 2013): 163–71.

6. D. F. Kripke, R. D. Langer, L. E. Kline, "Hypnotics' Association with Mortality or Cancer: A Matched Cohort Study," *British Medical Journal Open* 2, no. 1 (February 2012): e000850.

7. T. B. Huedo-Medina, I. Kirsch, J. Middlemass, M. Klonizakis, A. N. Siriwardena, "Effectiveness of Non-Benzodiazepine Hypnotics in Treatment of Adult Insomnia: Meta-Analysis of Data Submitted to the Food and Drug Administration," *British Medical Journal* 345 (December 2012): e8343.

8. D. Connelly, "Sales of Over-the-Counter Medicines in 2015 by Clinical Area and Top 50 Selling Brands," *Pharmaceutical Journal*, March 24, 2016.

9. Consumer Healthcare Products Association, "OTC Sales by Category 2013–2016," http://www.chpa.org/OTCsCategory.aspx, accessed May 2017.

10. Andy was a Football Association sponsorship executive back in 1998 who called me to sort out some better bedding for the English national squad at the 1998 World Cup in France. He still claims to this day that he started my career in sports.

11. A. W. McHill, E. L. Melanson, J. Higgins, E. Connick, T. M. Moehlman, E. R. Stothard, K. P. Wright Jr., "Impact of Circadian Misalignment on Energy Metabolism During Simulated Nightshift Work," *Proceedings of the National Academy of Sciences of the United States of America* 111, no. 48 (December 2, 2014): 17302–7.

12. F. Gu, J. Han, F. Laden, A. Pan, N. E. Caporaso, M. J. Stampfer, I. Kawachi, K. M. Rexrode, W. C. Willett, S. E. Hankinson, F. E. Speizer, E. S. Schernhammer, "Total and Cause-Specific Mortality of U.S. Nurses Working Rotating Night Shifts," *American Journal of Preventative Medicine* 48, no. 3 (March 2015): 241–52.

13. US Department of Energy, "Impact of Extended Daylight Saving Time on National Energy Consumption," October 2008.

14. J. Bidgood, "As Daylight Saving Starts, Some Ask: Why Fall Back at All?," *New York Times*, March 12, 2017.

15. B. T. Hansen, K. M. Sønderskov, I. Hageman, P. T. Dinesen, S. D. Østergaard, "Daylight Savings Time Transitions and the Incidence Rate of Unipolar Depressive Episodes," *Epidemiology* 28, no. 3 (May 2017): 346–53.

16. B. I. Omalu, S. T. DeKosky, R. L. Minster, M. I. Kamboh, R. L. Hamilton, C. H. Wecht, "Chronic Traumatic Encephalopathy in a National Football League Player, Part II," *Neurosurgery* 59, no. 5 (July 2005): 1086–92.

10. The Home Team: Sex, Partners, and the Modern Family

1. I first met Nick when he was working as a nutritionist at Blackburn Rovers FC with former Manchester United physiotherapist Dave Fevre. Nick then got me in to do some work with the squad when he was at Chelsea, and Carlo Ancelotti was the manager. Nick followed Carlo, who regarded him very highly, when he moved to Paris Saint-Germain. Sadly, Nick lost his life in tragic circumstances in France.

2. "Sleeping Difficulty In-Depth Report," *New York Times* Health Guide, http://www.nytimes.com/health/guides/symptoms /sleeping-difficulty/print.html, accessed May 2017.

3. S. Warner, G. Murray, D. Meyer, "Holiday and School-Term Sleep Patterns of Australian Adolescents," *Journal of Adolescence* 31, no. 5 (October 2008): 595–608.

4. E. Harbard, N. B. Allen, J. Trinder, B. Bei, "What's Keeping Teenagers Up? Prebedtime Behaviors and Actigraphy-Assessed Sleep over School and Vacation," *Journal of Adolescent Health* 58, no. 4 (April 2016): 426–32.

Acknowledgments

When I decided to start a family, I thought it was a good time to call it a day on trying to make it as a professional golfer, and so I joined the family furniture business. I could never have imagined back then that one day I would be asked by one of the leading international publishers to write a book about sleep.

So a big thank-you has to go out to everyone at Da Capo Lifelong Books, my publisher in the United States, and Penguin, my publisher in England, who played a part, with special thanks to Joel Rickett for supporting my approach and the need for a change in the way we look at sleep, and to Julia Murday for being so enthusiastic about the book and its contents, and putting together a launch program more fun than expected for the world of sleep.

Special thanks too go to my ghostwriter, Steve Burdett, who has taken all my experiences and encapsulated my passion to create a unique story about sleep that I hope will provoke comment and, most of all, redefine the approach of those who read it.

Thanks also to Patrick McKeown for giving up his time to talk about breathing, and to Rob Davies, a breathing-product innovator.

Just some of the people from my industry years need a mention: Peter Buckley, Morgan McCarthy, Patrick Newstead, the late Roger Head, Pam Johnson, Mark Bedford, Jeff Edis, and Alan Hancock. John Hancock and Jessica Alexander were instrumental in creating the first ever UK Sleep Council, where I met my sleep mentor, Chris Idzikowski.

Alex Ferguson, for his foresight way back in the late nineties, Dave Fevre, Lyn Laffin, Andy Oldknow of the FA, Gary Lewin, Rob Swire, and my dear friend the late Nick Broad all contributed to, if not kick-started, what has become my new career.

I had some of my best times developing a sleep retail business based in the heart of a resurgent Manchester, which provided some real city-living challenges that very much informed the R90 program, so thanks to Chris Lloyd, Howard and Judith Sharrock, Dave Simpson, Anna Litherland, Steve Silverstone, Brian McCall, Richard Locket, the late John Spencer, Flik Everett, Andy Nichol, Simon Buckley, Claire Turner, Kate Drewett, Roberto Simi, Zoe Vaughan Davies, Coby Langford, Darryl Freedman, Jason Knight, and John Quilter, plus so many more.

It was during this time that a new communications director joined Manchester United and chose to move to the same Northern Quarter street as my first shop. We remain friends to this day. Thank you for all your support: Phil Townsend and brother John.

A couple of other key Manchester moments really helped define the work I do today. The first came in 2009–10 when I got involved with British Cycling and the birth of Team Sky, whose success stories are clear for all to see, and never more so than over the summer of 2016, running into and during the Rio Olympic Games. So special thanks to Dave Brailsford, Matt Parker, Phil Burt, and Dr. Steve Baynes. The second key moment was consulting on Manchester City's new state-of-the-art training facility, so big thanks to Sam Erith for his support.

Without the support of my R90 product supply partners behind the scenes, I wouldn't have been able to complete many of my projects, so thanks to Icon Designs, Trendsetter, Acton & Acton, and Breasley.

For the future, thanks to Michael Torres of Shift Global Performance, my R90 partner in the United States, for all his and his team's support.

Of course, big thanks to my family, who have had to listen to endless talk about sleep. Perhaps, given that my father invented gasoline injection and traveled the world with his job in international motor racing, I should have been a racing driver, which might have made for more interesting conversation for them. But as new grandchildren appear and my family grows, my hope is that they've been listening to at least some of what I've been saying.